Biomedical Organizations

A Worldwide Guide to Position Documents

NOTES FOR PROFESSIONAL LIBRARIANS AND LIBRARY USERS

This is an original book title published by The Haworth Information Press®, an imprint of The Haworth Press, Inc. Unless otherwise noted in specific chapters with attribution, materials in this book have not been previously published elsewhere in any format or language.

CONSERVATION AND PRESERVATION NOTES

All books published by The Haworth Press, Inc., and its imprints are printed on certified pH neutral, acid-free book grade paper. This paper meets the minimum requirements of American National Standard for Information Sciences-Permanence of Paper for Printed Material, ANSI Z39.48-1984.

Biomedical Organizations

A Worldwide Guide to Position Documents

Dale A. Stirling

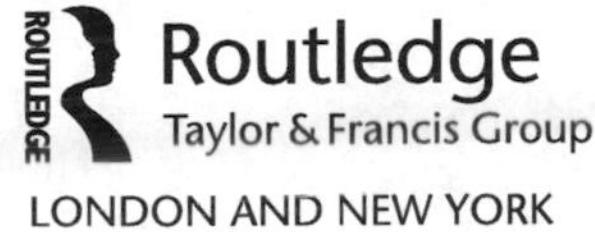

LONDON AND NEW YORK

First published 2006 by The Haworth Press, Inc.

2 Park Square, Milton Park, Abingdon, Oxfordshire OX14 4RN
605 Third Avenue, New York, NY 10017

Routledge is an imprint of the Taylor & Francis Group, an informa business

First issued in paperback 2020

Cover design by Jennifer M. Gaska.

Library of Congress Cataloging-in-Publication Data

Stirling, Dale A.
Biomedical organizations : a worldwide guide to position documents / Dale A. Stirling.
p. ; cm.
Includes bibliographical references and index.
ISBN-13: 978-0-7890-2297-4 (hc. : alk. paper)
ISBN-10: 0-7890-2297-4 (hc. : alk. paper)
ISBN-13: 978-0-7890-2298-1 (pbk. : alk. paper)
ISBN-10: 0-7890-2298-2 (pbk. : alk. paper)
1. Biomedical organizations—Policy statements. 2. Biomedical organizations—Policy statements—Indexes. I. Title.
[DNLM: 1. Health Services Administration. 2. Organizational Policy. 3. Organizations. W 84.1 S861b 2005]

R10.5.A3S85 2005
610'.68—dc22

2005009667

ISBN 978-0-7890-2298-1 (pbk)

CONTENTS

ABOUT THE AUTHOR

Dale A. Stirling, MA, has more than twenty years' experience as an environmental, natural resource, and public health issues historian, researcher, and writer. Mr. Stirling has authored numerous books, articles, reports, and conference papers. His articles have appeared in the *Practice Periodical of Hazardous, Toxic, and Radioactive Waste Management,* the *Bulletin of Bibliography,* and *Medical Reference Services Quarterly.* Prior to his involvement with Heritage North, a historical research firm specializing in environmental issues, natural resources, and public health research and writing, he was Senior Information Specialist at Intertox, Inc.

Foreword

Biomedical Organizations: A Worldwide Guide to Position Documents is a unique work that reviews over 1,000 medically related organizations worldwide representing a broad spectrum of medical services and practices. In a single source, Dale Stirling has compiled a comprehensive list of specific medical organizations as well as the process involved in the development of the position document. A discussion of an organization's stance on policy matters is included particularly as it relates to policy, position statements, and, in many cases, practice guidelines. These official statements reflect the opinions and consensus of the experts in their respective areas of medicine. Also listed are those organizations that do not have policy documents. As the complexity of medical practice evolves, the information currently available can be overwhelming. To utilize this information has often required tremendous amounts of personal research time. From the standpoint of a busy medical practitioner, this time is of the essence. Therefore, it is important to be able to refer to a single source for information on leading expert opinions and/or recommendations as reflected in their collective position statements, policies, procedures, and protocols. Physicians as well as paramedical personnel can benefit through the use of this work. Fellows, residents, interns, and even medical students can utilize this reference for better patient care and research. In addition, this publication is ideally suited as a unique composite reference text to be used in clinics and hospitals as well as medical and general libraries.

Mark Thoman, MD, FAAP, FACMT

Preface

There are more than 4,000 biomedical organizations worldwide representing the entire spectrum of medicine and medical practice. Accordingly, many of these organizations develop documents that reflect the collective position or opinion of their members on important issues of the day. These documents, most often referred to as position statements, are a unique resource not commonly consulted in the research process. They are the penultimate expression of a biomedical organization, as they represent the view of the association at a specific point in time, often based on the state of knowledge of a subject at a specific point in time. In 1996, while providing professional subconsulting services to a medical economics research firm, I realized that there was no single source of information about biomedical organization position documents. Therefore, over the next seven years I compiled documents and background information about the process of position document development. The results of that work are presented in this reference work. Of course, this book needed to satisfy more than one individual's curiosity or research needs. Therefore, a reasonable question is, what is the purpose of this book? The basic purpose of this book is to identify what biomedical organizations were thinking about in the early twenty-first century. More important, this book serves as a historical marker of a specific point in time. Organizations come and go; controversies and public opinion sway, change, and revert; however, a position regarding a specific topic or subject existed. Future researchers will have this guide to help them find out what that position was and what organization held it dear enough to have written a document. Aside from being a mere listing, this reference work also seeks to provide a historical account of position documents and their growth, continued use, and efficacy.

IDENTIFYING POSITION DOCUMENTS

The process of researching organization position statements was straightforward. An Internet search was conducted over a period of several years for biomedical organizations identified in the National Library of Medicine's Directory of Health Organizations Online (DIRLINE) and the MedNets.Com database of associations and societies. Although the emphasis was on organizations that represent biomedical professionals, selected and well-known health-related special interest groups (e.g., American Heart Association) that have research components were also included in the search. No geographic boundaries were placed on this search—every effort was made to review the Web sites of all biomedical organization with a Web presence. Nearly all foreign organization Web sites have at least an English translation of the organization's name. In some cases, a site map was provided in English. However, if the balance of the Web site was not in English, then that organization was not considered for this book. Once the Web site of the selected organization was located, a thorough review of the site was conducted to determine the presence of position statements or related documents. If no position statements were found during the online search, an e-mail was sent to the organization inquiring about the presence of position statements or lack thereof.

Four hundred to 500 e-mails were sent and approximately 30 percent responded. In those instances where no response was received, an additional Web site review was conducted. There are undoubtedly organizations with position statements not represented in this book. However, limitations had to be established and, therefore, if position statements were not found on a particular Web site or an organization did not respond to an e-mail request, then that organization is not included. Finally, hundreds of biomedical organizations are not represented here for the simple reason that they have not established any position documents—either because they are too small, do not have staff time and budget, or, more realistically, are state, regional, or local chapters of larger sister organizations and default to whatever positions the larger organizations have developed.

METHOD OF LISTING POSITION DOCUMENTS

The actual listing of position statements has been simplified such that only the most basic information is included—the biomedical organization's name, its Web site address, and an alphabetical listing of the organization's position documents. In general, position documents included in this book were published within the last ten years. No judgments were made about the accuracy, integrity, or appropriateness of any position documents. They speak for themselves. Therefore, it is up to the reader to make any value judgments. Similarly, no judgments were made about which biomedical organizations were included in the search. Some will argue that palliative and complementary and alternative medicine do not belong—the simple fact is that organizations exist to represent professionals in those fields; therefore, they deserve representation in this book. This guide to position documents also includes biomedical organizations that are tangentially related to core medical practices. For instance, councils, alliances, federations, and other organizations that operate on the periphery of a specific practice area are included. These organizations operate in support and promotion of practice specialists and often include trade groups.

In general, this work does not include evidence-based clinical practice guidelines or similar documents. Such guidelines are defined by the National Guideline Clearinghouse (1999) as "systematically developed statements to assist practitioner and patient decisions about appropriate health care for specific clinical circumstances." These guidelines are variously known as consensus opinions, medical care guidelines, practice parameters, and practice policies. It also does not include position documents of veterinary organizations. The reader should note that some biomedical organizations list position statements and practice guidelines concurrently, or define practice guidelines as position documents. Therefore, some biomedical organization entries include documents that are practice guidelines but are defined by the issuing organization as a position document.

INDEXING

With the idea that this reference work is a research tool, indexing was paramount. The index includes a primary heading followed by a list of the biomedical organization(s) that have issued position documents on that subject. The index is both topical and subject specific in nature. That is, it provides basic and extended indexing of topics. The entries are intended to provide the reader with a general feel for the topics covered in position documents generated by biomedical organizations. For instance, some readers will want to know which countries have biomedical organizations that have position documents—those are listed alphabetically by country name. Also, the subject index identifies medical practice areas—a reader can quickly check the index to determine the medical practice area of listed biomedical organizations (e.g., obstetrics, emergency medicine, or aerospace medicine). But the subject index is also quite specific in nature. That is, it provides a listing of medical subjects that are less about the general nature of medicine than about the core areas of interest specific to each biomedical organization. Therefore, the majority of these entries relate to issues such as abortion, gun control, terrorism, bicycle helmets, and all the other specific areas that these biomedical organizations have identified as being significant enough to warrant the creation of a position document.

Acknowledgments

I'm eternally grateful for the years of loving support and encouragement of my parents. Through highs and lows they've always had the vision to see the best of the future in me. For that I love them very much. For twenty-five years, my wife has put up with a multitude of side projects and concurrent writing assignments—from those poetic to those practical. I could not ask for a more loyal companion on the road to knowledge.

An Overview of Position Documents

POSITION DOCUMENTS DEFINED

A review of thousands of biomedical organization Web sites reveals that there is more than one type of position document. The following definitions are based on and abstracted from those developed by the International Pharmaceutical Federation (2001), Pennsylvania Medical Society (2000), and Society for Public Health Education (1982). For the purposes of this book, a position document is not related to the functioning of the organization (administrative, legal, financial, and educational) and does not provide clinical practice guidelines.

Discussion paper: A document that examines many factors relating to a specific topic and usually presents possible options for solutions or courses of action. The purpose of a discussion paper is to stimulate debate with a view to establishing an organization's position on a topic, thus making possible the drafting of a position or policy paper.

Position paper: A document that establishes the view of an organization on a specified date, based on the state of knowledge of the subject at that time. This document normally is developed in a situation where knowledge is developing rapidly or circumstances are changing. Position papers are often subject to continual review and are often time limited in scope. Eventually, however, with regular reviews, position papers often become policy papers.

Policy paper: A document that establishes an organization's current, firm policy on a specific subject. It is a document that the organization's members promote to other medical organizations and interested groups.

Resolution: "A resolution is the vehicle that conveys . . . a component society's proposal on a particular subject. Statements beginning with 'whereas' . . . include the introductory facts or circumstances which logically develop into a formal conclusion or the 'resolved portion.' The formal conclusion is the . . . 'resolved' portion of the resolution. The 'resolved' portion should stand alone as a complete and understandable statement. A resolution is also a statement that identifies and describes a health education issue and calls for specific action. Resolutions also serve an intermediary purpose as they often are the genesis of the more formal policy document development process" (National Association of County and City Health Officials, 1998).

Statement of principles or declarations: A document that sets out the position of an organization on a subject that has broad-based international implications but is not perceived as being directly related to the association's medical practice area.

THE HISTORICAL IMPERATIVE

A review of several thousand biomedical organization Web sites reveals that position documents are largely an American invention. Indeed, the majority of biomedical organizations in the United States maintain or have developed one or more position documents. Conversely, relatively few biomedical organizations outside the United States have developed position documents. The best sources of information about the genesis of biomedical organization documents are these organizations' own guidelines on position document development. According to the Society for Neuroscience (1999), "scientific societies exist for many purposes, one of which is to establish guidelines for responsible conduct within the field they represent." In most biomedical organizations, the authority and responsibility for establishing positions are more varied than organization policy, which is nearly always placed in the hands of the organization's board of directors. Therefore, proposed positions are sometimes submitted by members in good standing (Society for Public Health Education, 1982), by members in good standing in concert with a sponsoring entity (Ambulatory Pediatric Association, 2001), or by ad hoc committees (Society for Neuroscience, 1999). In some instances, the process is formal and requires an official application form for a new position paper (International Nurses Society on Addictions, 1999). Another impetus for position document development appears to be the cachet attached to establishing such documents. Because position documents impart an aura of scholarship to the issuing organization,

> it is recognized that governmental and non-governmental organizations, the wider scientific community, the media and the public are unlikely to be influenced by a society which has not taken a position on a particular topic when other . . . medical societies have done so. (British Toxicology Society, n.d., p. 2)

Finally, another impetus is legacy. Biomedical organizations are proud of their heritage and the place they occupy in their specific field. Therefore they have a vested interest in "shaping the major directions the field has taken over the years" (Leigh, 1987, p. 347). Still others desire to be authoritative in the face of controversy. The International Society for Clinical Densitometry (Leib et al., 2002) has cited "the need for authoritative positions in areas of controversy" (p. 5) and the British Academy of Emergency Medicine (Clangy, 2001) has stated, "position statements will be used to clarify the specialty's viewpoint in areas that range from the undisputed to the controversial" (p. 329).

Some biomedical organizations issue position documents as a means of establishing a track record on specific issues. For instance, the Ambulatory Pediatric Association (2001) states,

> it is essential that the organization also address public policy issues vital to child health. It is for this reason that the Board of Directors . . . has established this policy development process. APA policies will provide a historical record of the association's stance on a variety of child health related topics. (p. 1)

Biomedical organizations have differing methods of position document delivery. Many organizations post position documents only on their Web sites; however, other organizations publish their position documents in the official journal representing their organization, and then post them on their Web sites. Examples of this approach include the American College of Medical Toxicology *(Internet Journal of Medical Toxicology),* the American College of Occupational and Environmental Medicine *(Journal of Occupational and Environmental Medicine),* the British Academy of Emergency Medicine *(Emergency Medicine Journal),* and the Council on Learning Disabilities *(Learning Disability Quarterly).*

POSITION DOCUMENT EFFICACY

It seems natural to ask whether position documents are effective. A review of the sparse literature on the etiology of the position document provides few opinions. For instance, in reviewing a position statement on palliative care and euthanasia, the authors conclude that "the position paper seems to have attempted a compromise, in order to deal with the diversity of views" (Campbell and Huxtable, 2003, p. 182). The question of efficacy appears less important than the process of identifying an issue and preparing an appropriately related documented position. However, biomedical organizations pride themselves on their stance among peers; therefore, the development process is nearly always rigid and conforms to written guidelines. As one author states, "the value of any organization's position statement(s) is influenced by a multitude of factors (e.g., author's expertise, accuracy, evidence, opinion, etc.); thus, some degree of scrutiny is advised" (Strayer, 1996, p. 62). Perhaps the best assessment of the value of position documents was published by the Council on Learning Disabilities in 1987:

> The CLD board of trustees is confident that implementation of the recommendations made relative to each issue will result in significant improvements in the quality of services provided to individuals with learning disabilities. Board of trustee members look forward to engaging in the thoughtful discussion and debate with our fellow professionals that will inevitably be provoked by publication of the position statements. It is our contention that serious questions and problems currently confronting professionals in our field deserve nothing less. (Leigh, 1987, p. 348)

Some gauge of the efficacy of an organization's policy documents is its existence. Those that remain relevant are retained in the compendium of documents; those that are no longer relevant, or that have been superseded by newer versions, are retired and no longer cited. Regardless of the motivation for developing position documents, it is clear that biomedical organizations will continue to establish positions on a wide variety of topics. A sense of the importance of these documents is seen in a review of the literature of position documents (see Appendix B). In the past twenty years, more than fifty articles listing biomedical organization position documents have been published in the biomedical literature. Some organizations, such as AAOHN, ANNA, and ANA, regularly publish their latest position documents for the benefit of their members. Still others publish articles that announce revised or new position documents or describe the process of establishing an organization's position document.

Biomedical Organization Position Documents

Academy of Clinical Laboratory Physicians and Scientists
<http://depts.washington.edu/lmaclps>

Position Statement

- Exclusive Licenses for Diagnostic Tests

Academy of Hospice and Palliative Medicine
<http://www.aahpm.org>

Position Statements

- Ethics of Palliative Care Research
- Nutrition and Hydration
- Physician-Assisted Suicide

Academy of Managed Care Pharmacy
<http://www.amcp.org>

Position Statements

- Anticompetitive Pricing
- Any Willing Provider Legislation
- Collaborative Practice Agreements
- Direct-to-Consumer Advertising of Prescription Products
- Electronic Transfer of Prescription Information
- Formularies
- Interchange of Narrow Therapeutic Index Drugs
- Managed Health Care System Access to Electronically Transmitted Prescriptions
- Off-Label Use of Pharmaceuticals
- Patient Confidentiality
- Patient Rights and Responsibilities
- Prescription Drug Coverage
- Therapeutic Interchange

Policy Statements Adapted from AMCP Concept Papers

- Disease State Management
- Drug Names, Labels, and Packaging
- Drug Use Evaluation

- Managed Care Pharmacy Practice Residency Programs
- Pharmaceutical Care
- Pharmacist Role in Formulary Management
- Pharmacists' Cognitive Services
- Pharmacists' Role in Immunization
- Pharmacists' Role in Outcomes Research

Policy Statements Adapted from Other Pharmacy Organizations

- Code of Ethics for Pharmacists
- Conscientious Objection by Pharmacists to Certain Therapies
- Continuing Education for Pharmacists
- Ensuring Continuing Competence for Pharmacists
- Generic Drug Products
- Medication Administration by Pharmacists
- Needle Exchange Programs
- Pain Management and Support for Dying Patients
- The Pharmacist's Role in Detecting and Reporting Adverse Drug Reactions
- Preventing Medication Errors in Pharmacies and Managed Health Care Systems
- Public Funding for Pharmacy Residency Programs
- Tobacco and Tobacco Products
- Use of Drug Distribution Systems
- The Use of Pharmacy Technicians in Support of Managed Care Pharmacists

Position Statements

- Anticompetitive Pricing
- Any Willing Provider Legislation
- Collaborative Practice Agreements
- Compensation for Pharmaceutical Care Services
- Direct-to-Consumer Advertising
- The FDA-Proposed MedGuide Legislation
- Formularies
- Government-Mandated Private Sector Pharmacy Benefits
- Interchange of Narrow Therapeutic Index (NTI) Drugs
- Medicare Prescription Drug Coverage
- Off-Label Use of Pharmaceuticals
- Patient Confidentiality
- Patient Rights and Responsibilities
- Prescription Drug Coverage
- Prescription Drug Reimportation
- Therapeutic Interchange

Practice Policy Statements and Guidelines

- AMCP Supports the Use of a Federally Issued Unique Universal Identifier Number
- Application of Dispensing Criteria to All Providers
- Clinical Investigations in Children
- Communicating Drug and Device Recalls
- Consumer Information on Complementary and Alternative Medications
- Development of Performance Measures
- Diagnosis Inclusion on Prescriptions and Medication Orders
- Disease-Based Clinical Practice Guidelines
- Drug Abuse Programs
- Electronic Pharmacy Data Processes
- Elements of Quality Assessment
- Ensuring Drug Integrity and Stability
- Evidence-Based Advertising of Pharmaceuticals
- Health and Wellness Grants
- Health Care Team Approach to Optimal Therapeutic Outcomes
- Healthy People 2010
- Impaired Pharmacist Employment Waiver Requests
- Nontraditional Education
- Pharmacist Access to Patient Information
- Pharmacist Educational Advancement
- Pharmacist-Patient Communication
- Pharmacist Responsibility in the Drug Distribution Process
- Pharmacy CPT Codes
- Policy Collaboration to Achieve Optimal Patient Outcomes
- Professionalism and Professional Judgment
- Promotion and Certification of Pharmacy-Based Health Management Programs
- Restricted Distribution of Pharmaceuticals
- Standardized Pharmacy Benefit Cards
- State Pharmacy Practice Act Revisions
- Universal Health Care Provider Number

Academy of Medical-Surgical Nurses
<http://www.medsurgnurse.org>

Position Statement

- Mandatory Overtime

Academy of Psychosomatic Medicine
<http://www.apm.org>

Position Statements

- End-of-Life care
- Psychiatric Consultation Services for Medical/Surgical Patients

Aerospace Medical Association
<http://www.asma.org>

Position Papers

- Cardiac Conditions and Medical Tracking of Pilots in Acrobatic Flight
- Cockpit Resource Management

Key Resolutions

- Aggressive Airline Passengers
- Aircrew Fatigue
- Carry-on Luggage
- Health and Safety of Manned Commercial Space Flights
- Human Factors Training
- In-Flight Emergency Medical Kit
- In-Flight Medical Event Repository
- Laser Lights
- Medical Oxygen for Airline Passengers
- Smoking
- Uniformed Services University of the Health Sciences

Air and Surface Transport Nurses Association
<http://www.astna.org>

Position Papers

- Care of the Pediatric Patient During Interfacility Transfer
- Drug Testing for Flight Nursing
- Educational Recommendation for Nurses Providing Pediatric Emergency Care
- Flight Nurse Certification
- Flight Nurse Safety in the Air Medical Environment
- Improving Flight Nurse Safety in the Air-Medical Helicopter Environment
- Intravenous Conscious Sedation in Air Medical Transport
- Latex Allergy
- Mutual Recognition Model for Multistate Licensure

- Role of the Registered Nurse in Basic Life Support Air Transport
- Role of the Registered Nurse in the Prehospital Environment
- Staffing of Critical Care Air Medical Transport Services

Air Medical Physician Association
<http://ampa.org>

Position Statements

- Appropriateness of Air Medical Transport in Acute Coronary Syndromes
- Medical Condition List and Appropriate Use of Air Medical Transport
- Medical Direction and Medical Control of Air Medical Services

Alberta Dental Association and College
<http://www.abda.ab.ca>

Position Papers

- Dental Amalgam
- Dental Unit Waterline Contamination
- Providing Quality Dental Care for Your Company
- Providing Quality Dental Care for Your Employees

Alberta Medical Association
<http://www.albertadoctors.org/home>

Position Statements

- Abortion and Euthanasia
- AIDS/HIV
- Barer-Stoddart Report, Comments on
- Chelation Therapy
- Cost Containment
- Early Return to Work
- Goods and Services Tax
- Gun Control
- Health Care Costs
- Home Care
- Long-Term Care
- Member Advocacy
- Mental Health
- Mental Health Needs of the Elderly
- Mental Health Services, Children
- Midwifery

- Multicultural Health Care Delivery
- Prichard Report, Comments on
- Primary Medical Care
- Privacy of Personal Health Information
- Public Opinion
- Rainbow Report, Comments on
- Regionalization (Including Election of Regional Health Authorities)
- Reproductive Technologies
- Rural Medical Care
- Sexual Assault Protocol
- Sexual Exploitation—Response to Preliminary Report
- Smoking

American Academy of Addiction Psychiatry
<http://aaap.org>

Policy Statements

- Addressing Substance Abuse: A Priority in Health Care Reform
- Clean Needle and Syringe
- Legalization of Drugs
- Medical Use of Marijuana
- National Minimal Benefits Health Care Package
- Nicotine Dependence
- Office-Based Opioid Treatment
- Organ Transplantation
- Parity
- Professional Activities by Physicians with Restricted Medical Licenses
- Relationship Between Treatment and Self-Help
- Use of Illegal Substances by Pregnant Women

American Academy of Audiology
<http://www.audiology.org/index.php>

Position Statements

- Aged Persons with Hearing Impairment
- Audiologic Guidelines for the Diagnosis and Treatment of Otitis Media in Children
- Audiology Clinical Practice Algorithms and Statements
- Audiology: Scope of Practice
- Auditory Integration Training
- Cochlear Implants in Children

- Conflicts of Professional Interest
- Consensus Panel on Support Personnel in Audiology
- Ethics and the Use of Graduate Degrees
- Graduate Education
- Prepurchase Assessment Guideline for Amplification Devices
- The Professional Doctorate
- Role of the Audiologist in the Newborn Hearing Screening Program
- Use of Doctoral Degree Designators

American Academy of Child and Adolescent Psychiatry
<http://aacap.org>

Policy Statements

- Adolescent Pregnancy and Abortion
- Adolescent Pregnancy Prevention
- Apartheid
- Corporal Punishment in Schools
- Criteria for Clinical Privileges for Physician Members of Medical Staff
- Drug and Alcohol Screening
- Facilitated Communication
- Family Intervention in the Assessment and Treatment of Infants, Children, and Adolescents
- Governance of the Academy Web Site
- Guidelines for the Clinical Evaluation for Child and Adolescent Sexual Abuse
- HIV and Psychiatric Hospitalization of Children and Adolescents
- HIV and Youth
- Issues in Utilization Management
- Model for Minimum Staffing Patterns for Hospitals Providing Acute Inpatient Treatment for Children and Adolescents with Psychiatric Illnesses
- Placement of American Indian Children
- Position Paper on Substance Abuse Treatment and the Role of the Child
- Position Statement on Intelligence
- Position Statement on Newborn Infant Adoptions
- Prescribing Psychoactive Medication for Children and Adolescents
- Principles of Universal Access: Child and Adolescent Psychiatric Services
- Protecting Children Undergoing Abuse Investigations and Testimony

- Psychiatric Diagnostic Evaluations
- Psychotherapy as a Core Competence of Child and Adolescent Psychiatrists
- Restrictions on the Prescribing Practices of Child and Adolescent Psychiatrists by Managed Care Formularies
- The Role of Child and Adolescent Psychiatrists in Organized Systems of Care
- The Role of Child and Adolescent Psychiatrists in Reviewing Medical Necessity of Care
- Roles and Responsibilities of Child and Adolescent Psychiatry in the Field of Developmental Disabilities
- Screening Children for Lead: Guidelines for Children and Adolescent Psychiatrists
- Secretin in the Treatment of Autism
- Sexual Harassment
- Sexual Orientation and Civil Rights

American Academy of Clinical Toxicology
<http://www.clintox.org>

Position Statements

- Cathartics
- Gastric Lavage
- Gut Decontamination
- Ipecac Syrup
- Single-Dose Activated Charcoal
- Whole Bowel Irrigation

American Academy of Emergency Medicine
<http://aaem.org>

Position Statements

- Advanced Cardiac Life Support Course
- Advanced Trauma Life Support Course
- Due Process
- Emergency Medical Services
- Emergency Physician Credentialing
- FSMB Consensus Proposal
- Managed Care
- Mandatory Error Reporting
- Moonlighting/FSMB Recommendations

- Nondiscrimination between Practice Track and Residency-Trained EM Physicians
- Nondiscrimination of Practice Track versus Residency-Trained EM Physicians
- Nurse-to-Patient ED Staffing Ratios
- Performance of Emergency Screening Ultrasound Examinations
- Physician Assistants/Nurse Practitioners
- Physician-to-Patient ED Staffing Ratios
- The Role of Government in Securing Emergency Medical Care
- Unions in Emergency Medicine
- Use of Amiodarone in Refractory Pulseless VT/VF
- The Use of Intravenous Thrombolytic Therapy in the Treatment of Stroke

American Academy of Family Physicians
<http://aafp.org>

Health Policies

- Abortion
- Adolescent Health Care
- Advertising
- Aging
- Alcohol
- Ancillary Medical Personnel
- Area Health Education
- Assault Weapons
- Bicycle Helmet Laws
- Boxing
- Breast-feeding
- Capitation, Primary Care
- Case Manager, Definition
- Certificates of Added Qualification
- Certification
- Certification/Recertification, Definitions
- Certified Nurse Midwives
- Chelation Therapy
- Child Abuse
- Cigarettes
- Circumcision
- Clinical Proctoring
- Collaborative Practice Arrangements
- Community and Migrant Health Centers

- Complementary Practice
- Comprehensive Care
- Concurrent Care
- Confidentiality, Patient/Physician
- Confidentiality, Physician/Patient Communications
- Consultants/Backup
- Consultation, Definition
- Consultations/Referrals, Mandatory
- Continuing Medical Education
- Continuity of Care Definition
- Contraceptive Advice
- Corporal Punishment
- Correctional Health Care
- Council of Medical Specialty Societies
- Critical Care Medicine
- Diagnostic Screening
- Direct-to-Consumer Advertising
- Discrimination
- Disease State Management
- Documentation of Training and Experience
- Driver Education
- Drivers, Impaired, Drunk, or Drugged
- Driver's License
- Drugs
- Drunk Driving
- Economic Credentialing
- Education
- Education, Continuing Medical
- Education, Physician Retraining
- Elder Abuse
- Electrocardiography, Screening
- Emergency Medical Care
- Emergency Medical Services
- Endometrial Sampling, Screening
- Environment, Pollution of
- Equal Opportunity
- Essential Community Provider
- Ethics
- Excellence of Care
- Facility-Based Care
- Family
- Family Health Month

- Family Medicine Interest Groups
- Family Physician
- Family Practice
- Fees
- Female Genital Mutilation
- Firearms/Handguns
- Fluoridation of Public Water Supplies
- Fluoride
- Fragmentation of Care
- Freedom of Choice
- "Frontier Areas," Medical Care Roles
- Geriabuse
- Geriatrics
- Good Samaritan Law
- Government Encroachment in Medical Practice
- Handicapped Students, Participation in Physical Education
- Health Benefits
- Health Care
- Health Care Costs
- Health Care Delivery
- Health Care Insurance
- Health Centers
- Health Clinics
- Health Education
- Health Insurance
- Health Plans
- Health Workforce
- Hearing Impairment
- Home Health Care
- Homeless People
- Home Test Kits
- Hospice, Definition
- Hospital Accreditation
- Hospital Departments
- Hospitalization of Abused Children
- Hospital Medical Staff
- Hospital Privileges
- Hospitals
- Imaging Personnel
- Immunization Costs
- Impaired Persons, Participating in Sports
- Infant Health

- Integrated Practice Arrangements
- Laboratories
- Laboratory Referrals
- Laboratory Technicians
- Laetrile
- Legislative Activities
- Liaison Guidelines
- Licensure
- Licensure/Relicensure, Definitions
- Life-Sustaining Treatment
- Long-Term Care
- Long-Term Care Facilities
- Malpractice
- Managed Care
- Marijuana
- Maternal/Child Care
- Medicaid Services
- Medical Care
- Medical Identification
- Medical Informatics
- Medical Liability
- Medical Schools
- Medicare/Medicaid Abuses
- Medicare Reimbursement
- Membership
- Mental Health
- Midwives, Certified Nurse
- Migrant Health Care
- Military Service, Physician's Draft
- Minority Health Care
- Minority Students, Family Physicians as Role Models for
- National Health Service Corps
- Nicotine Addiction
- Nicotine Productions, Nonprescription
- Noise and Hearing Loss
- Nonphysicians Providers
- Nuclear Disaster Planning
- Nuclear Weapons
- Nurse Midwives, Certified
- Nurse Practitioners
- Nursing Profession
- Obstetrics

- Patient Care
- Patient-Centered Formularies
- Patient Discrimination
- Patient Responsibility for Follow-Up
- Patient Self-Referral
- Pediatric Patients and Emergency Care
- Peer Review
- Pharmaceutical Care
- Pharmacists
- Physician and Patient Relationships
- Physician Assistants
- Physician Profiling
- Physician-Sponsored Networks
- Physician Workforce Reform
- Physicians, Clinically Deficient
- Physicians, Impaired
- Point-of-Service Plans
- Political Action
- Population-Based Care Management
- Pre- and Postoperative Care
- Preceptorships
- Preventive Medicine
- Primary Care
- Primary Care Physician, Generic
- Primary Care Services for Limited Specialists
- Privileges
- Procedural Skills
- Professional Competence Evaluation
- Professional Medical Liability
- Proprietary Practices
- Quality, Definition
- Quality Health Care
- Quality Management in Patient Care
- Radiology Technicians
- Reeducation
- Referrals
- Regionalization/Networking
- Reimbursement
- Reproductive Decisions
- Research
- Resident Education, Discrimination
- Rural Health Care

- Safety
- Sex Education
- Sexually Transmitted Diseases
- Smoking, Tobacco
- Sports Medicine
- Standards of Care
- Steroids
- Student Education
- Students
- Substance Abuse
- Surgery
- Surgical Assistant Privileges
- Teaching, Physician Responsibility
- Teenage Pregnancy
- Telemedicine
- Television
- Tobacco and Smoking
- Transfer of Patient
- Utilization Review Programs
- Violence
- Women in Family Medicine
- Women's Health Care Issues
- Women's Health Specialty

Clinical Policy Statements

- Alternative Practice or Medicine
- Antibiotics
- Breast Cancer
- Cardiopulmonary Resuscitation
- Cervical Cancer, Screening for
- Chelation Therapy
- Cholesterol Screening, in Adults
- Circumcision
- Clinical Policies with Other Organizations
- Clinical Practices
- Complementary Practice or Medicine
- Electrocardiography, Screening
- Endometrial Sampling, Screening
- HIV Infection Statements and Policies
- Human Immunodeficiency Virus (HIV) Infection
- Immunization
- Laetrile

- Mammography
- Otitis Media
- Pap Test
- Periodic Health Examinations
- Steroids/Anabolic Androgenic, Use of
- Thimerosal in Vaccines
- Tuberculin Skin Testing, in Adults
- Vaginal Birth After Cesarean
- Vitamins

American Academy of Medical Acupuncture
<http://www.medicalacupuncture.org>

Position Statements
- Acupuncture Qualifications
- Definition of Acupuncture
- Needles and Devices
- Nonphysician Practitioners of Acupuncture

American Academy of Neurology
<http://www.aan.com/professionals>

Position Statements
- Animals in Research, Use of (unpublished)
- Assisted Suicide, Euthanasia, and the Neurologist
- Care and Management of Profoundly and Irreversibly Paralyzed Patients with Retained Consciousness and Cognition, Certain Aspects of
- Demented Patient, Ethical Issues in the Management of
- Ethical Issues in Clinical Research in Neurology
- Ethical Role of Neurologists in the AIDS Epidemic
- Expert Witness, Qualifications and Guidelines for the Physician (unpublished)
- Gun Control Position Statement (unpublished)
- Human Immunodeficiency Virus-Type 1 (HIV-1) Infection, Nomenclature, and Research Case Definitions for Neurologic Manifestations of Human Immunodeficiency Virus-Type 1 (HIV-1) in Neurologic Practice, Guidelines for Prevention of Transmission
- Palliative Care in Neurology
- Persistent Vegetative State Patient
- Physician Workforce in Neurology
- Power of Attorney for Health Care

American Academy of Nurse Practitioners
<http://aanp.org/default.asp>

Position Statements

- Advanced Practice Role
- Cost Effectiveness
- Nurse Practitioners' Authority
- Nurse Practitioners in Managed Care Organizations
- Prescriptive Authority
- Tobacco Fund
- Tobacco Use

American Academy of Ophthalmology
<http://aao.org>

Policy Statements

- Adult Strabismus
- Amblyopia Is a Medical Condition
- Color Codes for Topical Ocular Medications
- Eye Care in the Department of Veterans Affairs
- Frequency of Ocular Examinations
- Gifts to Physicians from Industry
- Glasses as a Medical Necessity
- Guidelines for Appropriate Referral of Persons with Possible Eye Diseases or Injuries
- Guidelines for Avoidance of Inadvertent Anticompetitive Conduct
- Laser Surgery
- Learning Disabilities, Dyslexia, and Vision
- Misinformation About Ophthalmology or the Academy
- Ophthalmic Care for Patients in Residential Centers
- Ophthalmic Care of the Medically Underserved
- Ophthalmologist's Duties Concerning Postoperative Care
- Policy for Academy Leaders
- Pretreatment Assessment: Responsibilities of the Ophthalmologist
- Protective Eyewear for Young Athletes
- Relationships with Other Organizations
- The Role of Ophthalmology and the Ophthalmologist
- Tissue Procurement for Corneal Transplantation
- Use of Unapproved Lasers and Software for Refractive Surgery
- Vision Requirements for Driving
- Vision Screening for Infants and Children

American Academy of Optometry
<http://www.aaopt.org>

Position Papers

- Comanagement
- Extended Wear
- Monovision
- Orthokeratology
- Ultraviolet
- Vision, Learning, and Dyslexia

American Academy of Oral and Maxillofacial Pathology
<http://www.aaomp.org>

Policy Statement

- Tissue Submission

American Academy of Oral and Maxillofacial Radiology
<http://www.aaomr.org>

Position Papers

- Characteristics of an Oral and Maxillofacial Radiology Department
- Imaging of the Temporomandibular Joint
- Implant Imaging
- Infection Control

American Academy of Orthopedic Surgeons
<http://aaos.org>

Position Statements

- All-Terrain Vehicles
- Anabolic Steroids to Enhance Athletic Performance
- Animals in Biomedical Research
- Banning Antipersonnel Land Mines
- Containing the Cost of Orthopedic Implants
- Credentialing in the Use of Specialized Instrumentation in Orthopedics
- Delineation of Clinical Privileges in Orthopedic Surgery
- Early Return to Work Programs
- Family Violence
- Fee "Unbundling" and Uniform Definitions for Surgical Procedures
- Financing of Graduate Medical Education
- Firearms Violence

- Health Care Coverage for Children at Risk
- Health Care Plan Accountability
- Helmet Use by Motorcycle Drivers and Passengers and Bicyclists
- Helmet Use in Skiing
- Hip Fracture in Seniors: A Call for Health System Reform
- Improving America's Trauma Care System
- Injuries from In-Line Skating
- In-Office Diagnostic Imaging Studies by Orthopedic Surgeons
- Managed Care in Workers' Compensation
- Medical and Surgical Procedure Patents
- Medical Error/Patient Safety Reporting Systems
- Medical Savings Accounts
- Medicare Joint Replacement Demonstration Project
- Medicare Payments to New Physicians
- Need for Daily Physical Activity
- Osteoporosis as a National Public Health Priority
- Physician DRGs
- Power Lawn Mower Safety
- Power Snow Thrower/Blower Safety
- Prescription Drug Coverage Under Medicare
- Prevention of Hip Fractures
- Principles of Medicare Reform
- Professional Liability: Tort Reform
- Prompt Payment of Physician Claims
- Reimbursement of the First Assistant at Surgery in Orthopedics
- Relationships Between Health Care Plans and Trauma Systems
- Reprocessed Single-Use Devices
- Risks of Shoulder and Elbow Injury from Participation in Youth Baseball
- Safety Belts
- School Screening Programs for the Early Detection of Scoliosis
- Scope of Orthopedic Practice in Managed Care Arrangements
- Sledding Safety
- Smoking and the Musculoskeletal System
- Sports and Recreational Programs for Physically Disabled People
- Surgical Care of the Lower Extremities
- Telemedicine, Computers, and the Internet
- Trampolines and Trampoline Safety
- Twenty-Four-Hour Coverage Concept
- Use of Breakaway Bases in Preventing Recreational Baseball and Softball Injuries
- Use of Knee Braces

American Academy of Orthotists and Prosthetists
<http://www.oandp.org>

Position Statements

- On Ethical Conduct of Orthotic and Prosthetic Practitioners
- On Practitioners Giving Testimony
- On the Minimum Education Essentials and Credentialing for Providers of Comprehensive Orthotic and Prosthetic Services
- On the Provision of Custom Fabricated, Fitted, and/or Designed Orthoses and Prostheses
- Orthotic and Prosthetic Services
- State Licensure

American Academy of Otolaryngologic Allergy
<http://www.aaoaf.org>

Policy Statements

- Allergy Evaluation
- Chemical Sensitivity
- Food Allergy
- Inhalant Allergy (Allergic Rhinitis)
- Organic Inhalants
- Otolaryngologic Allergy

American Academy of Pain Medicine
<http://www.painmed.org>

Position Statements

- Acute Pain and Cancer Pain
- Basic Principles of Ethics for the Practice of Pain Medicine
- Consent for Chronic Opioid Therapy
- Definitions Related to the Use of Opioids for the Treatment of Pain
- Long-Term Controlled Substances Therapy for Chronic Pain, Sample Agreement
- The Necessity for Early Evaluation and Treatment of the Chronic Pain Patient
- Quality Care at the End of Life
- Undergraduate Medical Education on Pain Management, End-of-Life Care, and Palliative Care
- The Use of Opioids for the Treatment of Chronic Pain

American Academy of Pediatric Dentistry
<http://www.aapd.org>

Oral Health Policies

- Adolescent Oral Health
- Alternative Restorative Treatment
- Baby Bottle Tooth Decay/Early Childhood Caries
- Beverage Vending Machines in Schools
- Breast-feeding
- The Dental Home
- Dietary Recommendations for Infants, Children, and Adolescents
- Early Childhood Caries: Unique Challenges and Treatment Options
- Emergency Oral Care for Children
- Hospitalization for Dental Care of Infants and Children
- Immunization of Infants, Children, and Adolescents
- Infection Control
- Intraoral and Perioral Piercing
- Minimizing Occupational Health Hazards Associated with Nitrous Oxide
- Operating Room Access for Pediatric Dental Care
- Oral and Maxillofacial Surgery for Infants, Children, and Adolescents
- Oral Habits
- Oral Health Care Programs for Infants, Children, and Adolescents
- Prevention of Sports-Related Orofacial Injuries
- Revised Hospital Staff Membership
- Revised Third-Party Reimbursement of Fees Related to Dental Sealants
- Third-Party Reimbursement of Dental Costs Related to Congenital Orofacial Anomalies
- Third-Party Reimbursement of Medical Costs Related to Sedation/General Anesthesia
- Tobacco Use
- The Use of a Caries Risk Assessment Tool for Infants, Children, and Adolescents
- The Use of Deep Sedation and General Anesthesia in the Pediatric Dental Office
- The Use of Fluoride

American Academy of Pediatrics
<http://www.aap.org>

Policy Statements

- Access to Pediatric Emergency Medical Care

- Administration of the Third Dose of Oral Poliomyelitis Vaccine at Six to Eighteen Months of Age
- Adolescent Assault Victim Needs: A Review of Issues and a Model Protocol
- Adolescent Pregnancy
- Adolescents and Anabolic Steroids: A Subject Review
- Adolescents and Human Immunodeficiency Virus Infection: The Role of the Pediatrician in Prevention and Intervention
- Adolescent's Right to Confidential Care When Considering Abortion
- Advanced Practice in Neonatal Nursing
- Age for Routine Administration of the Second Dose of Measles-Mumps-Rubella Vaccine
- Age Limits of Pediatrics
- Alcohol Use and Abuse: A Pediatric Concern
- All-Terrain Vehicle Injury Prevention
- All-Terrain Vehicles
- Alternative Routes of Drug Administration—Advantages and Disadvantages
- Aluminum Toxicity in Infants and Children
- Ambient Air Pollution: Respiratory Hazards to Children
- Amenorrhea in Adolescent Athletes
- Antitrust Policy
- Appropriate Boundaries in the Pediatrician-Family-Patient Relationship
- Asbestos Exposure in Schools
- Athletic Participation by Children and Adolescents Who Have Systemic Hypertension Atlantoaxial Instability in Down Syndrome: Subject Review
- Auditory Integration Training and Facilitated Communication for Autism
- Basic Life Support Training in School
- Behavioral and Cognitive Effects of Anticonvulsant Therapy
- Bicycle Helmets
- Breast-feeding and the Use of Human Milk
- Calcium Requirements of Infants, Children, and Adolescents
- Camphor Revisited: Focus on Toxicity
- Cardiac Dysrhythmias and Sports
- Care Coordination
- Care of Adolescent Parents and Their Children
- Changing Concepts of Sudden Infant Death Syndrome
- Chemical-Biological Terrorism and Its Impact on Children

- Child in Court: A Subject Review
- Child Life Services
- Children, Adolescents, and Advertising
- Children, Adolescents, and Television
- Children and Fireworks
- Children in Pickup Trucks
- Children with Health Impairments in Schools
- Cholesterol in Childhood
- Circumcision Policy Statement
- Climatic Heat Stress and the Exercising Child and Adolescent
- Clioquinol (Iodochlorhydroxyquin, Vioform) and Iodoquinol (Diiodohydroxyquin): Blindness and Neuropathy
- Combination Vaccines for Childhood Immunization
- Condom Availability for Youth
- Confidentiality in Adolescent Health Care
- Consensus Report for Regionalization of Services for Critically Ill or Injured Children
- Consent for Medical Services for Children and Adolescents
- Constipation in Infants and Children: Evaluation and Treatment
- Contraception and Adolescents
- Controversies Concerning Vitamin K and the Newborn
- Cord Blood Banking for Potential Future Transportation: Subject Review
- Corporal Punishment in Schools
- Counseling the Adolescent About Pregnancy Options
- Critique of the Final Report—Graduate Medical Education National Advisory Committee
- Culturally Effective Pediatric Care
- Developmental Issues for Young Children in Foster Care
- Diagnostic Imaging of Child Abuse
- Directory of Overseas Service Opportunities for Pediatricians
  Disclosure of Illness Status to Children and Adolescents with HIV Infection
- Distinguishing Sudden Infant Death from Child Abuse Fatalities
- Does Bed Sharing Affect the Risk of SIDS?
- Doman-Delacato Treatment of Neurologically Handicapped Children
- Do Not Resuscitate Orders in Schools
- Drowning in Infants, Children, and Adolescents
- Drug-Exposed Infants
- Drugs for Pediatric Emergencies
- Echocardiography in Infants and Children

- Education of Children with Human Immunodeficiency Virus Infection
- Efforts to Reduce the Toll of Injuries in Childhood Require Expanded Research
- Emergency Physician and the Office-Based Pediatrician: An EMSC Team
- Emergency Preparedness for Children with Special Health Care Needs
- Enhancing the Racial and Ethnic Diversity of the Pediatric Workforce
- Environmental Tobacco Smoke: A Hazard to Children
- Ethanol in Liquid Preparations Intended for Children
- Ethical Issues in Surrogate Motherhood
- Ethics and the Care of Critically Ill Infants and Children
- Evaluation and Medical Treatment of the HIV Exposed Infant
- Evaluation and Preparation of Pediatric Patients Undergoing Anesthesia
- Evaluation of the Newborn with Developmental Anomalies of the External Genitalia
- Eye Examination and Vision Screening in Infants, Children, and Young Adults
- Facilities and Equipment for the Care of Pediatric Patients in a Community Hospital
- Families and Adoption: The Pediatrician's Role in Supporting Communication
- Female Genital Mutilation
- Fetal Alcohol Syndrome and Alcohol-Related Neurodevelopmental Disorders
- Fetal Therapy—Ethical Considerations
- 55 Miles per Hour Maximum Speed Limit
- Financing of Substance Abuse Treatment for Children and Adolescents
- Firearms and Adolescents
- Firearms-Related Injuries Affecting the Pediatric Population
- Fitness, Activity, and Sports Participation in the Preschool Child
- Folic Acid for the Prevention of Neural Tube Defects
- Forgoing Life-Sustaining Medical Treatment in Abused Children
- General Principles in the Care of Children and Adolescents with Genetic Disorders and Their Chronic Health Conditions
- Generic Prescribing, Generic Substitution, and Therapeutic Substitution
- Gifts to Physicians from Industry

- Gonorrhea in Prepubertal Children
- Graduate Medical Education and Pediatric Workforce Issues and Principles
- Guidance for Effective Discipline
- Guidelines and Levels of Care for Pediatric Intensive Care Units
- Guidelines for Developing Admission and Discharge Policies for Pediatric Intensive Care
- Guidelines for Expert Witness Testimony in Medical Liability Cases
- Guidelines for Home Care of Infants, Children, and Adolescents with Chronic Disease
- Guidelines for Monitoring and Management of Pediatric Patients During and After Sedation for Diagnostic and Therapeutic Procedures
- Guidelines for Ophthalmologic Examinations in Children with Juvenile Rheumatoid Arthritis
- Guidelines for Pediatric Cardiology Diagnostic and Treatment Centers
- Guidelines for Pediatric Emergency Care Facilities
- Guidelines for the Administration of Medication in School
- Guidelines for the Diagnosis and Management of Asthma
- Guidelines for the Ethical Conduct of Studies to Evaluate Drugs in Pediatric Populations
- Guidelines for the Evaluation of Sexual Abuse of Children: Subject Review
- Guidelines for the Pediatric Cancer Center and Role of Such Centers in Diagnosis and Treatment
- Guidelines for the Pediatric Preoperative Anesthesia Environment
- Guidelines for Urgent Care in School
- Guidelines on Forgoing Life-Sustaining Medical Treatment
- Guiding Principles for Managed Care Arrangements for the Health Care of Newborns, Infants, Children, Adolescents, and Young Adults
- Hazards of Child Labor
- Health Appraisal Guidelines for Day Camps and Resident Camps
- Health Care for Children and Adolescents in Detention Centers, Jails, Lockups, and Other Court-Sponsored Residential Facilities
- Health Care for Children of Farmworker Families
- Health Care for Children of Immigrant Families
- Health Needs of Homeless Children and Families
- Health Supervision for Children with Down Syndrome
- Health Supervision for Children with Marfan Syndrome
- Health Supervision for Children with Neurofibromatosis

- Health Supervision for Children with Sickle Cell Diseases and Their Families
- Health Supervision for Children with Turner Syndrome
- Hepatitis C Virus Infection
- Home, Hospital, and Other Non-School-Based Instruction for Children and Adolescents Who Are Medically Unable to Attend School
- Homosexuality and Adolescence
- Horseback Riding and Head Injuries
- Hospital Discharge of the High-Risk Neonate—Proposed Guidelines
- Hospital Record of the Injured Child and the Need for External Cause-of-Injury Codes
- Hospital Stay for Healthy-Term Newborns
- How Pediatricians Can Respond to the Psychosocial Implications of Disasters
- Human Immunodeficiency Virus/Acquired Immunodeficiency Syndrome Education in Schools
- Human Immunodeficiency Virus and Other Blood-Borne Viral Pathogens in the Athletic Setting
- Human Immunodeficiency Virus Screening
- Human Milk, Breast-feeding, and Transmission of Human Immunodeficiency Virus
- Hypoallergenic Infant Formulas
- Identification and Care of HIV-Exposed and HIV-Infected Infants, Children, and Adolescents in Foster Care
- Immunization of Adolescents
- Immunizations for Native American Children
- Impact of Music Lyrics and Music Videos on Children and Youth
- Implementation of the Immunization Policy (S94-26)
- Implementation Principles and Strategies for Title XXI
- "Inactive" Ingredients in Pharmaceutical Products: Update
- Inappropriate Use of School "Readiness" Tests
- Indications for Management and Referral of Patients Involved in Substance Abuse
- Infant Methemoglobinemia: The Role of Dietary Nitrate
- Infants with Anencephaly as Organ Sources: Ethical Considerations
- Infection Control in Physicians' Offices
- Informed Consent, Parental Permission, and Assent in Pediatric Practice
- Inhalant Abuse
- Initial Medical Evaluation of an Adopted Child

- Initiation or Withdrawal of Treatment for High-Risk Newborns
- Injuries Associated with Infant Walkers
- Injuries in Youth Soccer: A Subject Review
- Injuries Related to "Toy" Firearms
- In-Line Skating Injuries in Children and Adolescents
- Insurance Coverage of Mental Health and Substance Abuse Services for Children and Adolescents
- Integrated School Health Services
- Intensive Training and Sports Specialization in Young Athletes
- Investigation and Review of Unexpected Infant and Child Deaths
- Iron Fortification of Infant Formulas
- Issues in Newborn Screening
- Issues in the Application of the RBRVS System to Pediatrics: A Subject Review
- Issues of Confidentiality in Adoption: The Role of the Pediatrician
- Issues Related to Human Immunodeficiency Virus Transmission in Schools, Child Care, Medical Settings, the Home, and Community
- Knee Brace Use by Athletes
- Learning Disabilities, Dyslexia, and Vision: A Subject Review
- Liability and Managed Care
- Managed Care and Children with Special Health Care Needs: A Subject Review
- Marijuana: A Continuing Concern for Pediatricians
- Maternal Phenylketonuria
- Measles Immunization in HIV-Infected Children
- Media Education
- Media Violence
- Medicaid Policy Statement
- Medical Concerns in the Female Athlete
- Medical Conditions Affecting Sports Participation
- Medical Home
- Medical Home Statement Addendum: Pediatric Primary Health Care
- Medically Indicated Home, Hospital, and Other Non-School-Based Instruction
- Medical Necessity for the Hospitalization of the Abused and Neglected Child
- Medical Staff Appointment and Delineation of Pediatric Privileges in Hospitals
- Meningococcal Disease Prevention and Control Strategies for Practice-Based Physicians

- Mitral Valve Prolapse and Athletic Participation in Children and Adolescents
- Neonatal Anesthesia
- Neonatal Drug Withdrawal
- Newborn and Infant Hearing Loss: Detection and Intervention
- Newborn Screening Fact Sheets
- Newborn Screening for Congenital Hypothyroidism: Recommended Guidelines
- Noise: A Hazard for the Fetus and Newborn
- Nondiscrimination in the Care of Pediatric Patients
- Nondiscrimination in the Delivery of Pediatric Health Care
- Office-Based Counseling for Injury Prevention
- Oral and Dental Aspects of Child Abuse and Neglect
- Organized Athletics for Preadolescent Children
- Palliative Care for Children
- Parental Leave for Residents and Pediatric Training Programs
- Participation in Boxing by Children, Adolescents, and Young Adults
- PCBs in Breast Milk
- Pediatric Care Recommendations for Free-Standing Urgent Care Facilities
- Pediatric Physician Profiling
- Pediatric Services for Infants and Children with Special Health Care Needs
- Pediatric Workforce Statement
- Pediatricians and Childhood Bereavement
- Pediatricians and the "New Morbidity"
- Pediatrician's Responsibility for Infant Nutrition
- Pediatrician's Role in Advocating Life-Support Courses for Parents
- Pediatrician's Role in Community Pediatrics
- Pediatrician's Role in Development and Implementation of an Individual Education Plan and/or an Individual Family Service Plan
- Pediatrician's Role in Disaster Preparedness
- Pediatrician's Role in Family Support Programs
- Pediatrician's Role in Helping Children and Families Deal with Separation and Divorce
- Pediatrician's Role in the Prevention of Missing Children
- Perinatal Care at the Threshold of Viability
- Perinatal Human Immunodeficiency Virus Testing
- Personal Watercraft Use by Children and Adolescents
- Physician's Role in Coordinating Care of Hospitalized Children
- Planning for Children Whose Parents Are Dying of HIV/AIDS

- Policy on the Development of Immunization Tracking Systems
- Population-to-Pediatrician Ratio Estimates: A Subject Review
- Possible Association of Intussusceptions with Rotavirus Vaccination
- Practical Significance of Lactose Intolerance in Children: Supplement
- Precautions Concerning the Use of Theophylline
- Precertification Process
- Prenatal Genetic Diagnosis for Pediatricians
- Prenatal Visit
- Prescription Drug Advertising Direct to the Consumer
- Prevention and Management of Pain and Stress in the Neonate
- Prevention of Hepatitis A Infections: Guidelines for Use of Hepatitis A Vaccine and Immune Globulin
- Prevention of Lyme Disease
- Prevention of Medication Errors in the Pediatric Inpatient Setting
- Prevention of Pneumococcal Infections, Including the Use of Pneumococcal Conjugate and Polysaccharide (Technical Report) Vaccines and Antibiotic Prophylaxis
- Prevention of Poliomyelitis: Recommendations for Use of Only Inactivated Poliovirus Vaccine for Routine Immunization
- Prevention of Respiratory Syncytial Virus Infections: Indications for the Use of Palivizumab and Update on the Use of RSV-IGIV
- Prevention of Sexual Harassment in the Workplace
- Prevention of Unintentional Injury Among American Indian and Alaska Native Children
- Principles and Guidelines for Early Hearing Detection and Intervention Programs
- Principles of Child Health Care Financing
- Privacy Protection of Health Information: Patient Rights and Pediatrician Responsibilities
- Professional Liability Coverage for Residents and Fellows
- Prolonged Infantile Apnea
- Promotion of Healthy Weight-Control Practices in Young Athletes
- Protective Eyewear for Young Athletes
- Provision of Educationally Related Services for Children and Adolescents with Chronic Diseases and Disabling Conditions
- Provision of Related Services for Children with Chronic Disabilities
- Psychosocial Risks of Chronic Health Conditions in Childhood and Adolescence
- Public Disclosure of Private Information About Victims of Abuse
- Qualifications and Utilization of Nursing Personnel Delivering Health Services in Schools

- Race/Ethnicity, Gender, Socioeconomic Status—Research Exploring Their Effects on Children
- Radon Exposure: A Hazard to Children
- Reappraisal of Lytic Cocktail/Demerol, Phenergan, and Thorazine for the Sedation of Children
- Reassessment of the Indications for Ribavirin Therapy in Respiratory Syncytial Virus Infections
- Recommendations for Preventive Pediatric Health Care
- Recommendations for the Prevention of Pneumococcal Infections, Including the Use of Pneumococcal Conjugate Vaccine (Prevnar), Pneumococcal Polysaccharide Vaccine, and Antibiotic Prophylaxis
- Recommendations for the Use of Live Attenuated Varicella Vaccine
- Recommendations on Extracorporeal Membrane Oxygenation
- Recommended Childhood Immunization Schedule—United States, January-December 2000
- Recommended Timing of Routine Measles Immunization for Children Who Have Recently Received Immune Globulin Preparations
- Reducing the Number of Deaths and Injuries from Residential Fires
- Reducing the Risk of Human Immunodeficiency Virus Infection Associated with Illicit Drugs
- Reimbursement for Medical Foods for Inborn Errors of Metabolism
- Relationship Between Pertussis Vaccine and Central Nervous System Sequelae
- Religious Objections to Medical Care
- Report on the Management of Primary Vesicoureteral Reflux in Children
- Residency Training and Continuing Medical Education in School Health
- Revised CDC Guidelines for Isolation Precautions in Hospitals: Implications for Pediatrics
- Revised Guidelines for Prevention of Early Onset Group B Streptococcal Infection
- Revised Indications for the Use of Palivizumab and Respiratory Syncytial Virus Immune Globulin Intravenous for the Prevention of Respiratory Syncytial Virus Infections
- Risk of Injury from Baseball and Softball in Children 5 to 14 Years of Age
- Risk of Ionizing Radiation Exposure to Children: A Subject Review
- Role of Home-Visitation Programs in Improving Health Outcomes for Children and Families

- Role of Pediatrician in Recognizing and Intervening on Behalf of Abused Women
- Role of Schools in Combating Substance Abuse
- Role of the Nonphysician Provider in the Delivery of Pediatric Health Care
- Role of the Nurse Practitioner and Physician Assistant in the Care of Hospitalized Children
- Role of the Pediatrician in Implementing the Americans with Disabilities Act
- Role of the Pediatrician in Prescribing Therapy Services for Children with Motor Disabilities
- Role of the Pediatrician in Prevocational and Vocational Education of Children and Adolescents with Developmental Disabilities
- Role of the Pediatrician in Rural EMSC
- Role of the Pediatrician in Youth Violence Prevention in Clinical Practice and at the Community Level
- Role of the Primary Care Pediatrician in the Management of High-Risk Newborn Infants
- Routine Evaluation of Blood Pressure, Hematocrit, and Glucose in Newborns
- Safeguards Needed in Transfer of Patient Data
- Safe Transportation of Newborns at Hospital Discharge
- Safe Transportation of Premature and Low Birth Weight Infants
- Safety in Youth Ice Hockey: The Effects of Body Checking
- School Bus Transportation of Children with Special Needs
- School Health Assessments
- School Transportation Safety
- Scope of Health Care Benefits for Infants, Children, and Adolescents, and Young Adults Through Age 21 Years
- Screening and Diagnosis of Autism
- Screening Examination of Premature Infants for Retinopathy of Prematurity
- Screening for Retinopathy in the Pediatric Patient with Type 1 Diabetes Mellitus
- Screening Infants and Young Children for Developmental Disabilities
- Selecting and Using the Most Appropriate Car Safety Seats for Growing Children
- Selecting Appropriate Toys for Young Children: The Pediatrician's Role
- Severe Invasive Group A Streptococcal Infections: A Subject Review

- Sexual Assault and the Adolescent
- Sexuality, Contraception, and the Media
- Sexuality Education of Children and Adolescents with Developmental Disabilities
- Shaken Baby Syndrome: Inflicted Cerebral Trauma
- Skateboard Injuries
- Smokeless Tobacco: A Carcinogenic Hazard to Children
- Snowmobiling Hazards
- Soy Protein-Based Formulas: Recommendations for Use in Infant Feeding
- Statement of Principle of the Provisional Committee on International Child Health
- Statement on Pediatric Fellowship Training
- Sterilization of Minors with Developmental Disabilities
- Strength Training, Weight and Power Lifting, and Body Building by Children and Adolescents
- Suicide and Suicide Attempts in Adolescents
- Surfactant Replacement Therapy for Respiratory Distress Syndrome
- Surveillance of Pediatric HIV Infection
- Swimming Programs for Infants and Toddlers
- Targeted Tuberculin Testing and Treatment of Latent Tuberculosis Infection
- The Teenage Driver
- Testing for Drugs of Abuse in Children and Adolescents
- Therapy for Children with Invasive Pneumococcal Infections
- Timing of Elective Surgery on the Genitalia of Male Children with Particular Reference to the Risks, Benefits, and Psychological Effects of Surgery and Anesthesia
- Tobacco, Alcohol, and Other Drugs
- Tobacco-Free Environment: An Imperative for the Health of Children and Adolescents
- Toxic Effects of Indoor Molds
- Trampolines at Home, School, and Recreational Centers
- Transfer of Drugs and Other Chemicals into Human Milk
- Transition of Care for Adolescents with Special Needs
- Transmissible Spongiform Encephalopathies: A Review for Pediatricians
- Transporting Children with Special Health Care Needs
- Treating Tobacco Use and Dependence
- Treatment Guidelines for Lead Exposure in Children
- Treatment of Neurologically Impaired Children Using Patterning
- Triathlon Participation by Children and Adolescents

- Type 2 Diabetes in Children and Adolescents
- Ultraviolet Light: A Hazard to Children
- Unapproved Uses of Approved Drugs
- Universal Access to Good-Quality Education and Care of Children from Birth to 5 Years
- Update on Timing of Hepatitis B Vaccination for Premature Infants and for Children with Lapsed Immunizations
- Update on Tuberculosis Skin Testing of Children
- Use and Abuse of the Apgar Score
- Use of Chaperones During the Physical Examination of the Pediatric Patient
- Use of Codeine- and Dextromethorphan-Containing Cough Remedies in Children
- Use of Fruit Juice in the Diets of Young Children
- Use of Inhaled Nitric Oxide
- Use of Physical Restraint Interventions for Children and Adolescents in the Acute Care Setting
- Use of Psychoactive Medication During Pregnancy and Possible Effects on the Fetus and Newborn
- Use of Whole Cow's Milk in Infancy
- Varicella Vaccine Update
- Why Supplemental Security Income Is Important for Children with Disabilities
- WIC Program

American Academy of Periodontology
<http://www.perio.org>

Position Papers

- Chemical Agents for Control of Plaque and Gingivitis
- Current Understanding of the Role of Microscopic Monitoring, Baking Soda, and Hydrogen Peroxide
- Diabetes and Periodontal Diseases
- Diagnosis of Periodontal Diseases
- Epidemiology of Periodontal Diseases
- Lasers in Periodontics
- Oral Features of Mucocutaneous Disorders
- The Pathogenesis of Periodontal Diseases
- Periodontal Considerations in the HIV-Positive Patient
- Periodontal Considerations in the Management of the Cancer Patient

- Periodontal Disease As a Potential Risk Factor for Systemic Diseases
- Periodontal Diseases of Children and Adolescents
- Periodontal Management of Patients with Cardiovascular Diseases
- Periodontal Regeneration
- Peroxide in the Treatment of Periodontal Disease
- The Potential Role of Growth and Differentiation Factors in Periodontal Regeneration
- The Role of Controlled Drug Delivery for Periodontitis
- The Role of Supra- and Subgingival Irrigation in the Treatment of Periodontal Diseases
- Sonic and Ultrasonic Scalers in Periodontics
- Supportive Periodontal Therapy
- Systemic Antibiotics in Periodontics
- Tissue Banking and Periodontal Bone Allografts
- Tobacco Use and the Periodontal Patient
- Treatment of Gingivitis and Periodontitis

American Academy of Physician Assistants
<http://www.aapa.org>

Position Statements

- Complementary and Alternative Medicine 2000
- A Continuing Medical Education and the Physician Assistant Profession
- Drunk Driving, the Legal Criteria
- End-of-Life Decision Making
- Entitlement Funding for Physician Assistant Education
- Ethics in Managed Care
- Flexibility As a Hallmark of the PA Profession: The Case Against Specialty Certification
- Guidelines for Amending Hospital Staff Bylaws
- Guidelines for Ethical Conduct by the Physician Assistant Profession (Adopted 2000)
- Guidelines for State Regulation of Physician Assistants
- Guidelines for the Physician Assistant Serving As an Expert Witness
- Health Care System Reform
- Human Immunodeficiency Virus Infection
- Human Immunodeficiency Virus in the 90s
- Immunizations in Children and Adults
- Managed Health Care and Rural America

- Physician Assistant Impairment
- Physician Assistants and Clinical Practice Guidelines
- Physician Assistants and Innovative Solutions for Rural Hospitals
- Physician Assistants As Medicaid Managed Care Providers
- Physician Assistants As Medical Review Officers
- Physician Assistants' Roles in Health Promotion and Disease Prevention
- Professional Competence
- Report of the AAPA Task Force on Unlicensed Medical Graduates
- Rural Health Clinics

Policy Briefs

- Antimicrobial Resistance
- Diagnosis and Management of HIV-Positive Patients
- Federal Funding for Embryonic Stem Cell Research
- Genetic Testing in Clinical Practice
- HIV Infection and Public Health Surveillance
- Partner Notification, Contact Tracing, and the HIV Epidemic

American Academy of Psychiatry and the Law
<http://aapl.org>

Position Statement

- Death Penalty

American Academy of School Psychology
<http://espse.ed.psu.edu/spsy/aasp/aasp.ssi>

Position Statement

- Identification of Learning Disabilities

American Academy of Sleep Medicine
<http://www.aasmnet.org>

Position Statements

- AASM Standards "Technologist Staffing"
- Indications for the Clinical Use of Unattended Portable Recording for the Diagnosis of Life Insurance Risk Assessment in Patients with Obstructive Sleep-Disordered Breathing
- Role and Qualifications of Technologists Performing Polysomnography
- Sleep-Related Breathing Disorders
- Use of Animals in Sleep Research
- Use of Gamma Hydroxybutyrate in the Treatment of Narcolepsy

American Association for Geriatric Psychiatry
<http://www.aagpgpa.org>

Position Statements

- Access to Psychiatric Care for Patients with Alzheimer's Disease and Other Dementia
- The Clinical Roles and Functions of the Geriatric Psychiatrist
- End-of-Life Care
- Family and Caregiver Counseling in Dementia: Medical Necessity
- Formulary Choices and Restrictions
- Psychotherapeutic Medication in the Nursing Home

American Association for Medical Transcription
<http://www.aamt.org/scriptcontent/index.cfm>

Position Statement

- Quality Assurance

American Association for Mental Retardation
<http://aamr.org>

Position Statements: Systems

- Direct Support Professionals
- Prevention
- Research
- Service Coordination
- Waiting List

Position Statements: Rights

- Advocacy
- Criminal Justice
- Guardianship
- Human and Civil Rights
- Inclusion
- Protection
- Self-Determination

Position Statements: Life in the Community

- Aging
- Behavioral Supports
- Early Intervention
- Education
- Family Support
- Health Care

- Housing
- Individual supports
- Sexuality
- Spirituality
- Transportation

American Association for Pediatric Ophthalmology and Strabismus
<http://aapos.org>

Position Statements

- Aphakic Glasses
- Criteria for Screening Premature Infants for ROP
- Learning Disorders (Dyslexia)
- Medical Need for Glasses
- Refraction As Part of the Eye Exam
- Sensorimotor Exam
- Vision Screening for Infants and Children

Policy Statements

- Adult Strabismus Surgery: A Joint Position Statement Issued by AAO and the AAPOS
- Amblyopia Is a Medical Condition: A Joint Position Statement Issued by AAO and the AAPOS
- Aphakic Glasses
- Glasses As a Medical Necessity: A Joint Position Statement Issued by AAO and the AAPOS
- Learning Disorders (Dyslexia)
- Medical Necessity of Adult Strabismus Surgery: A Position Statement Issued by AAPOS
- Medical Need for Glasses
- Vision Screening for Infants and Children
- Vision Therapy for Learning Disabilities

American Association of Cardiovascular and Pulmonary Rehabilitation
<http://www.aacvpr.org>

Position Statements

- Cardiac Rehabilitation As Secondary Prevention
- Cardiac Rehabilitation Services: A Scientific Evaluation
- Efficacy of Risk Factor Intervention and Psychosocial Aspects of Cardiac Rehabilitation
- Scientific Basis of Pulmonary Rehabilitation

American Association of Clinical Endocrinologists
<http://www.aace.com>

Position Statements

- Obesity
- Subclinical Hypothyroidism During Pregnancy

American Association of Colleges of Nursing
<http://www.aacn.nche.edu>

Position Statements

- Assistive Personnel to the Registered Nurse
- The Baccalaureate Degree in Nursing As Minimal Preparation for Professional Practice
- Building Capacity Through University Hospital and University School of Nursing Partnerships
- Certification and Regulation of Advanced Nursing Practice
- Defining Scholarship for the Discipline of Nursing
- Distance Technology in Nursing Education
- Diversity and Equality of Opportunity
- Educational Mobility
- Education and Practice Collaboration
- Education for Nurses in Administrative Roles
- Faculty Shortages in Baccalaureate and Graduate Nursing Programs
- Hallmarks of the Professional Nursing Practice Environment
- Indicators of Quality in Research
- Interdisciplinary Education and Practice
- Licensure of International Students
- Nursing Education's Agenda for the 21st Century
- Nursing Research
- Strategies to Reverse the New Nursing Shortage
- Substance Abuse
- Violence As a Public Health Problem

American Association of Community Psychiatrists
<http://www.comm.psych.pitt.edu>

Position Papers

- Housing Options for Individuals with Serious and Persistent Mental Illness
- Interface and Integration with Primary Care Providers
- Involuntary Outpatient Commitment
- Persons with Mental Illness Behind Bars

- Postrelease Planning
- President's New Freedom Commission
- Program Competencies in a Comprehensive Continuous Integrated System of Care for Individuals with Co-occurring Psychiatric and Substance Disorders
- Representative Payeeships
- Standards for Quality Management in Implementing Public Sector Managed Care Systems

American Association of Critical Care Nurses
<http://www.aacn.org>

Position Statements

- Assuring Quality Health Care for the United States
- Financial Constraints
- Maintaining Patient-Focused Care in an Environment of Nursing Staff Shortages and Mandatory Overtime
- Role of the Critical Care Nurse
- Use of Animals in Research Funded by AACN Grants

American Association of Dental Examiners
<http://www.aadexam.org>

Position Statements

- The Elimination of the Dental and Dental Hygiene Clinical Licensure Examinations As a Requirement for Initial Licensure
- The Impact of the Elimination of the Use of Human Subjects in the Clinical Licensure Process by 2005

American Association of Electrodiagnostic Medicine
<http://www.aaem.net>

Position Statements

- Appropriate Payors for Carpal Tunnel Syndrome
- Billing for Same-Day Evaluation and Management and Electrodiagnostic Testing
- Credentialing of Physicians As Electrodiagnostic Medicine Consultants
- Educational Guidelines for Electrodiagnostic Training Programs
- Electrodiagnostic Testing of Pregnant Women
- Expert Witness Testimony
- Explanatory Statement: Mixed Nerve Conduction Studies: CPT™ Code 95904

- Guidelines for Establishing a Quality Assurance Program in an Electrodiagnostic Laboratory
- Guidelines for Ethical Behavior Relating to Clinical Practice Issues in Electrodiagnostic Medicine
- Inappropriate Requirement of Hard Copy Needle EMG for Reimbursement
- Inappropriate Requirement of Hard Copy of Nerve Conduction Study for Reimbursement
- Job Descriptions for Electrodiagnostic Technologists
- Qualifications of Physiatrists to Perform Electrodiagnostic Studies
- Recommended Educational Requirements for the Practice of Electrodiagnostic Medicine
- Recommended Policy for Electrodiagnostic Medicine
- Referral Guidelines for Electrodiagnostic Medicine Consultations
- Responsibilities of an Electrodiagnostic Technologist
- Role of Electrodiagnostic Technologists in the Operating Room
- Technologists Conducting NCSs and SEPs Independently to Be Reviewed by a Physician at a Later Time
- Who Is Qualified to Practice Electrodiagnostic Medicine?

American Association of Endodontists
<http://www.aae.org>

Position Statements

- Lasers in Dentistry
- Latex Allergies
- Paraformaldehyde-Containing Endodontic Filling and Sealing Materials

American Association of Gynecologic Laparoscopists
<http://aagl.org>

Position Statements

- Credentialing Guidelines for Operative Endoscopy
- Medical Necessity of Surgical Assistants at Laparscopic Surgery

American Association of Healthcare Administrative Management
<http://www.aaham.org>

Position Papers

- Charity Care Policy
- Medicare Secondary Payer (MSP) Screening
- Observation Outpatient Services

- OIG's Compliance Guidance for Small Physician Practices
- Third-Party Code of Conduct
- Third-Party Medical Billing Compliance
- Transfer of an Acute Care Patient to, from, and Within the Hospital

American Association of Health Plans
<http://www.ahip.org>

Issues of Interest

- Access/Cost
- ADA
- ADEA
- Affirmative State Legislation
- Antidiscrimination Laws
- Antitrust
- Care Management
- Children's Health
- Chronic Care
- Civil Rights
- Claims Regulation
- Class-Action Lawsuits
- Clinical Care Initiatives
- Clinical Trials
- ERISA
- Fiduciary Duty
- Genetics
- Guaranty Funds
- Health Entities Working Group
- Health Reserves
- HMO Model Act
- Long-Term Care
- Malpractice Reform
- Market Conduct Issues
- Mental Health
- NAIC Issues
- Patient Protection
- Pharmacy Model Act
- Preemption
- Prescription Drugs
- Prevention
- Privacy and HIPAA
- Privacy/Security

- Provider Contracting/Relations
- Public Programs
- Quality/Patient Safety
- Regulatory Framework Task Force
- Regulatory Reengineering
- Risk-Based Capital
- Senior Issues
- Small-Group Market Reform
- Utilization Review
- Women's Health

American Association of Medical Dosimetrists
<http://www.medicaldosimetry.org>

Position Statements
- Credentialing
- Education
- Medical Errors

American Association of Neurological Surgeons
<http://www.aans.org>

Position Statements
- Bone Dowels from Humans
- Placebo Surgery
- Placement of Intracranial Pressure Monitors by Midlevel Practitioners in Neurotrauma and Emergency Neurosurgical Care
- Use of Cervical Decompression for Chronic Fatigue Syndrome

American Association of Occupational Health Nurses
<http://www.aaohn.org>

Position Statements
- AAOHN/ACOEM Joint Statement on Confidentiality
- Confidentiality of Health Information
- Delivery of Occupational and Environmental Health Services
- Emergency Medical Technicians, Including Paramedics, in the Workplace
- Licensed Practical Nurse in Occupational Health
- Natural Rubber Latex Sensitivity
- The Occupational Health Nurse As a Case Manager
- Occupational Health Surveillance
- Use of Automatic External Defibrillators

Advisories

- Accident Investigation
- Adult Immunizations
- Americans with Disabilities Act
- Antitrust Considerations for Professionals
- Automatic External Defibrillator Intervention Program
- Best Practices in an Occupational Health and Safety Program: Voluntary Protection Program
- Case Management
- Confidentiality
- Consultant Practice in Occupational Health
- Cost Benefits and Cost-Effectiveness Analyses
- Developing Clinical Guidelines or Protocols for Practice
- Employee Health Records: Requirements, Retention, and Access
- Environmental Health: Expanding Dimensions of Practice
- The Family Medical Leave Act
- Getting Results with Psychiatric Fitness for Duty Exams
- Implementing Occupational and Environmental Health Services in the International Sector
- Integrated Health System Strategies
- Managing Professional Risk in Occupational and Environmental Health Nursing Practice
- Multistate Practice
- Nurse Practitioners in Occupational and Environmental Health
- Over-the-Counter Medications
- Providing Expert Testimony
- Understanding Certification
- Work Fitness Impairment Evaluation in Occupational and Environmental Health

American Association of Public Health Dentistry
<http://aaphd.org>

Policy Statements

- Ethics
- National Health Reform
- Primary Care

Resolutions

- Community Water Fluoridation
- Oral Health Services for Older Americans
- Pit and Fissure Sealants
- Placement of Dental Sealants by Dental Hygienists

- Smokeless Tobacco
- Taxing Employee Health Care Benefits
- Tobacco Cessation, Prevention, and Control
- Transmissible Diseases

Position Papers

- Access to Dental Care
- Community and School Water Fluoridation
- Control of Transmissible Diseases in Dental Practice
- The Future of Dental Public Health Report
- A Half-Century of Community Water Fluoridation in the United States
- Periodontal Disease in America: A Personal and National Tragedy
- A Research Agenda for Dental Public Health

American Association of Spinal Cord Injury Nurses
<http://www.aascin.org>

Position Statements

- Access to Health Care
- Advanced Practice Nurses
- Health Care Reform
- Medical Rehabilitation Insurance Benefits
- Nursing Education and Research
- The Peranesthesia Patient with a Do-Not-Resuscitate Advance Directive
- Prevention of Transmission of Blood-Borne Pathogens
- Registered Nurse in the Management of Patients Receiving IV
- Registered Nurse Utilization of Unlicensed Assistive Personnel
- Resolution in Support of a National Child Safety Lock Law
- The Role of Tuberculosis Prevention and Control
- Sedation for Short-Term Therapeutic, Diagnostic, or Surgical Procedures
- Unlicensed Assistive Personnel in Home Care Settings
- The Use of Placebos for Pain Management in Patients with Cancer
- Violence As a Leading Cause of Spinal Cord Injury

American Board of Internal Medicine
<http://www.abim.org>

Position Statements

- Access to Health Care: Educational Portfolio—What Is the Profession's Responsibility?
- Attending Physicians: Your Role in Evaluating Residents

- Caring for the Dying
- Geriatric Medicine
- Guidelines and Criteria for the ABIM General and Subspecialty Internal Medicine Research Pathway
- Guide to Awareness and Evaluation of Humanistic Qualities
- Guide to Evaluation of Residents in Internal Medicine
- Mini-Clinical Evaluation Exercise: Guidelines and Forms
- Project Professionalism
- Promoting Medical Interviewing Skills in Internal Medicine
- Recertification: Continuous Professional Development Program
- Residents: Evaluating Your Clinical Competence
- Resource Document for Subspecialty Program Directors: Clinical Competence Guidelines

American Board of Surgery
<http://www.absurgery.org>

Position Statements/Policy Issues
- ABS Diplomate and Examination Statistics
- Changes in CME Requirements for Subspecialty Recertification
- Continuing Medical Education Requirements
- Creation of an Independent Vascular Surgery Board
- Graduate Surgical Education: Current Trends, Future Directions
- Recertification in General Surgery and Subspecialties

American College Health Association
<http://www.acha.org>

Policy Statements
- ACHA Nondiscrimination Policy
- Antibias/Antiviolence Statement
- Cultural Competency Statement
- Internet Resolution

American College of Allergy, Asthma and Immunology
<http://acaai.org>

Position Statement
- Administration of Immunotherapy Outside of the Prescribing Allergist Facility

American College of Cardiology
<http://www.acc.org>

Policy and Position Statements

- Access to Cardiovascular Care
- Ambulatory Blood Pressure Monitoring: Position Statement
- Athletes
- Aviation
- Beta-Blockers/Adrenergic Beta-Antagonist
- Cardiac Angiography Without Cine Film
- Catheterization
- Chelation Therapy
- Chest Discomfort, Approaches to the Early Triage of Patients with
- Cholesterol Management
- Drug Industry
- Early Defibrillation
- Heart Rate Variability for Risk Stratification of Life-Threatening Arrhythmia
- Industry Relations
- In-Hospital Cardiac Monitoring of Adults for Detection of Arrhythmia
- Interventional Catheterization Procedures and Cardiothoracic Surgical Consultation
- Nuclear Cardiology Services
- Physician Workforce Issues
- Preventive Cardiology and Atherosclerotic Disease
- Radiographic Devices by Cardiologists
- Same-Day Surgical Admission

American College of Clinical Pharmacy
<http://www.accp.com>

Position Statements

- Collaborative Drug Therapy Management by Pharmacists
- Critical Care Pharmacy Services
- Drug Use in the Elderly
- Economic Evaluations of Clinical Pharmacy Services
- Evidence of the Economic Benefit of Clinical Pharmacy Services
- Guidelines for Pharmacoeconomic Research Fellowships
- Pharmacists and the Pharmaceutical Industry: Guidelines for Ethical Interactions
- Prospectus on the Economic Value of Clinical Pharmacy Services

American College of Emergency Physicians
<http://acep.org>

Issue Papers

- BAC Reporting
- Documentation Guidelines
- EMS Personnel Expanded Scope of Practice
- GME Funding
- Payment for Screening Exams
- Physician Assistants and Nurse Practitioners
- Practice Expense
- Prudent Layperson Federal Legislation
- Prudent Layperson Status
- Prudent Layperson Version
- Reassignment
- Risk Management

Policy Resource and Education Papers

- Background Regarding Gifts to Emergency Physicians from the Biomedical Industry
- Circadian Rhythms and Shift Work
- "Do Not Attempt Resuscitation" Orders in the Out-of-Hospital Setting
- The Emergency Physician and Patient Confidentiality: A Review
- Equipment for Ambulances
- Evaluation and Management of the Sexually Assaulted or Sexually Abused Patient
- Evaluation and Treatment of Minors: Reference on Consent
- Guidelines for Ambulance Diversion
- Guidelines for Credentialing and Delineation of Clinical Privileges in Emergency Medicine
- Guidelines for the Role of EMS Personnel in Domestic Violence
- Guidelines for Undergraduate Education in Emergency Medicine
- Health Care Guidelines for Cruise Ship Medical Facilities
- Management of Observation Units
- Medical Direction of Interfacility Patient Transfers
- Medical Direction of Prehospital Emergency Medical Services
- Military Prehospital Care and Emergency Medical Service Systems
- Motor Vehicle Safety: Current Concepts and Challenges for Emergency Physicians
- Out-of-Hospital 12-Lead ECG
- Physician Medical Direction of EMS Education Programs
- Recognition and Management of Elder Abuse

- Report on Preparedness of the Emergency Department for the Care of Children
- Resource Utilization in the Emergency Department: The Duty of Stewardship
- Use of Intravenous TPA for the Management of Acute Stroke in the Emergency Department
- Use of Peak Expiratory Flow Rate Monitoring for the Management of Asthma in Adults in the Emergency Department
- Verification of Endotracheal Tube Placement
- Voluntary Guidelines for Out-of-Hospital Practices

American College of Epidemiology
<http://www.acepidemiology2.org>

Policy Statements

- Epidomiology and Minority Population
- Ethics Guidelines
- Health Data Control, Access, and Confidentiality
- Sharing Data from Epidemiologic Studies

American College of Medical Genetics
<http://www.acmg.net>

Policy Statements

- Alzheimer's Disease, Consensus Statement on Use of Apolipoprotein E Testing for
- BRCA-1 Mutation in Ashkenazi Jewish Women, Statement on Population Screening for
- Breast and Ovarian Cancer
- Canavan Disease, Carrier Testing for
- Colon Cancer, Genetic Testing for
- Cystic Fibrosis Carrier Screening, Laboratory Standards and Guidelines for Population-Based
- Down Syndrome, Statement on Nutritional Supplements
- Duty to Recontact
- Evaluation of the Newborn with Single or Multiple Congenital Anomalies: A Clinical Guide
- Expert Witness Testimony for the Specialty of Medical Genetics, Guidelines for
- Factor V Leiden Mutation Testing, Consensus Statement on
- FISH2: FISH Technical and Clinical Assessment of: An ACMG/ASHG Position Statement. I: Technical Considerations

- Folic Acid and Pregnancy
- Folic Acid: Statement on Fortification and Supplementation
- Fragile X, Technical Standards and Guidelines for
- Fragile X Syndrome, Policy Statement on Diagnostic and Carrier Testing
- Gene Patents and Accessibility of Gene Testing
- Genetic Counseling in Advanced Paternal Age
- Genetics and Managed Care
- Genetic Testing in Adoption
- Genetic Testing in Children and Adolescents
- Informed Consent for Medical Photographs
- Measurement and Use of Total Plasma Homocysteine
- Multiple-Marker Screening in Pregnant Women, Statement on
- Multiple-Marker Screening in Women 35 and Older, Position Statement on
- Newborn Hearing Screening, Statement on Universal
- Prader-Willi and Angelman Syndromes, Diagnostic Testing for
- Preventing Unfair Discrimination Based on Genetic Disease Risk
- Principles of Screening
- Sequence Variations, Recommendations for Standards for Interpretation of
- Storage and Use of Genetic Materials
- Tandem Mass Spectrometry in Newborn Screening
- Uniparental Disomy

American College of Medical Physics
<http://www.acmp.org>

Policy Statements

- Definition of a Qualified Medical Physicist
- Diagnostic Radiology: Patient Dose and Entrance Skin Exposures
- Federal Regulatory Responsibilities for Medical Devices
- Image Interpretation, Production, and Quality
- Licensure for Medical Physicists
- Manufacturer-Provided Physics Services
- Medical Dosimetrist
- Medical Physics Services
- Professional Nature of Medical Physics
- Radiation Safety Officer
- Radioactive Materials and Patient Safety
- Reimbursement for the Services of Qualified Professional Medical Physicists

American College of Medical Quality
<http://acmq.org>

Professional Policies

- Appeals of Determinations Not Establishing Medical Necessity
- Application of Clinical Ethics in Medical Decision Making
- Backing of Laws That Foster the Admission of Medical Errors
- Collaboration on Clinical Guideline Development and Improvement
- Compliance with the Medical Review Process
- Confidentiality of Peer Review Information
- Cost-Benefit Analysis in Health Care
- Definition and Application of Experimental or Investigational Medical Services and Supplies
- Definition and Application of Medical Necessity
- Definition and Documentation Required to Support Skilled versus Custodial Care
- Definition of Clinical Quality Improvement
- Definition of Medical Quality
- Development and Usage of Practice Parameters for Medical Quality Decision Making
- Disclosure of Financial Interest in Prescribed Medical Products and Services
- Documentation
- Economic Credentialing
- The Effect of the Medical Review Process on the Clinical Practice of Medicine
- Financial Incentives Which Impact Upon Medical Decision Making
- Gag Clauses
- Independent Practitioners
- Language Barriers in Physician-Patient Communication
- Limiting Health Care Benefits
- The Medical Decision-Making Process
- Medical Expert Consulting/Testifying
- Medical Information Availability to the Public
- Medical School Education in Medical Quality Management
- Medical Treatment over the Internet
- Physician Advisor Credentialing
- Physician-Assisted Suicide
- Physician Credentialing
- Physician Peer Review
- Physician Self-Referral
- The Provision of Specialty Medical Care

- Report Cards/Profiling and Outcome Data
- The Role of Physicians in Promoting Patient Safety
- The Role of Prevention in Medical Quality Management
- Standard of Care
- Standards of Medical Quality Review Systems
- Tobacco

American College of Medical Toxicology
<http://www.acmt.net>

Position Statements
- Dietary Supplements
- Hospital Privileges for Physicians Practicing Medical Toxicology
- Interpretation of Urine Analysis for Cocaine Metabolites
- Material Safety Data Sheets
- Medication Errors and Adverse Drug Reactions or Events
- Poison Center Medical Directors
- The Role of a Medical Toxicologist in the Treatment of Alcohol Withdrawal Syndrome

American College of Nurse-Midwives
<http://acnm.org>

Position Statements
- Adolescent Health Care
- The Appropriate Use of Technology in Childbirth
- Breast-feeding
- The Certified Nurse-Midwife/Certified Midwife As First Assistant at Surgery
- CNM and CMs As Primary Care Providers/Case Managers
- Collaborative Management in Midwifery Practice
- Continuing Competency Assessment
- Definition of a CNM/Practice
- The Ethics of Continuing Education
- Expansion of Midwifery Practice
- Female Circumcision
- Health Care/Managed Care Reform
- Immunization Status of Women and Their Families
- Independent Midwifery Practice
- Intrapartum Nutrition
- Joint Statement of Practice Relations Between Obstetrician/Gynecologists and Certified Nurse-Midwifes Mandatory Degree Requirement

- Latex Allergy
- Midwifery Care of Women Planning a Vaginal Birth After Cesarean
- Midwifery Education
- Minority Affairs
- Quality Management in Midwifery Care
- Reproductive Choices
- Safeguarding Maternal and Infant Health
- Statement on HIV/AIDS
- Universal Access to Care for Women and Infants
- Universal Access to Health Care
- Violence Against Women

American College of Occupational and Environmental Medicine
<http://acoem.org>

Position Statements

- Alternative Medical Care
- Confidentiality of Medical Information in the Workplace
- Consensus Statement for Confidentiality of Employee Health Information
- Dissemination of Scientific Information Regarding the Health of Workers
- Environmental Responsibility
- Epidemiologic Basis for an Occupational and Environmental Policy on Environmental Tobacco Smoke
- Financing of Health Care for the AMA
- Genetic Screening in the Workplace
- Mandatory HIV Testing of Health Care Workers
- Medical Surveillance in the Workplace
- Microcurrent Electrical Neuromuscular Stimulation and Low-Energy Laser
- Multiple Chemical Sensitivities: Idiopathic Environmental Intolerance
- Occupational Noise-Induced Hearing Loss
- Particulate Matter Standards
- Pesticides and Children
- Potential Adverse Human and Environmental Health Impacts of Chlorinated Chemicals
- Radon Exposure
- Role of the Occupational Physician in Enhancing Productivity
- Telemedicine
- Use of Contact Lenses in an Industrial Environment

- Women's Health and the Environment
- Workers' Compensation Reform

American College of Osteopathic Emergency Physicians
<http://acoep.org/index.html>

Practice Policies

- Emergency Department Telephone Advice
- Emergency Department Ultrasound
- Emergency Medicine Practice Characteristics
- Rapid-Sequence Intubation
- The Role of Emergency Physicians in Preventive Medicine
- The Role of Physician Extenders in Emergency Departments

American College of Physicians
<http://www.acponline.org>

Featured Papers

- Background Paper: The Case for Graduate Medical Education As a Public Good
- Beyond MICRA: New Ideas for Liability Reform
- Confidentiality of Electronic Medical Records
- Direct-to-Consumer Advertising for Prescription Drugs
- Estimates of the Impact of Selected Medicare Changes
- Fairness and Equity for International Medical Graduates in the United States
- Firearms Injury Prevention
- Illegal Drug Abuse and National Drug Policy
- Inner-City Health Care
- Insurance Reform in a Voluntary System
- Medical Savings Accounts
- Medicare Private Contracting
- A National Health Workforce Policy
- Physician-Run Health Plans and Antitrust
- Physicians and Joint Negotiations
- Physician Workforce and Graduate Medical Education
- Reforming Medicare: Adapting a Successful Program to Meet New Challenges
- The Role of the Future General Internist Defined
- Strategies for Incremental Expansion of Access to Care: Steps to Universal Coverage

- The Urban Health Penalty: New Dimensions and Directions in Inner-City Health Care
- Voluntary Purchasing Pools

American College of Preventive Medicine
<http://www.acpm.org>

Public Policy Statements

- Folic Acid Fortification of Grain Products in the U.S. to Prevent Neural Tube Defects
- Needle Exchange Programs to Reduce Drug-Associated Morbidity and Mortality
- Strengthening Motor Vehicle Occupant Protection Laws

American College of Prosthodontics
<http://www.prosthodontics.org>

Position Statement

- Specialty Reimbursement

American College of Radiology
<http://www.acr.org/s_acr/index.asp>

Professional and Public Policy Statements

- Abdominal Radiological Examinations of Women of Childbearing Age and Potential
- ACR Endorsement of the American Registry of Diagnostic Medical Sonography
- ACR-NEMA Digital Imaging and Communications Standards
- American Registry of Radiological Technologists
- Biological Effects of Radiation
- Cardiovascular Technologist: Essentials and Guidelines of an Accredited Educational Program
- Continuing Education and Competence
- Credentialing and Training
- Criteria for the Use of Water-Soluble Iodinated Contrast Agents for Intravascular Injections
- Curietherapy
- Diagnostic Medical Sonographers: Essentials and Guidelines of an Accredited Educational Program
- Diagnostic Sonographer/Vascular Technologist: Scope of Practice
- Disposal of Low-Level Radioactive Waste

- Drugs: ACR Support of Conjoint Effort to Facilitate New Drug Approval
- Drugs and Equipment
- Effect of Physician Workforce Restructuring
- Essentials of the Intersociety Commission for Accreditation of Vascular Laboratories, Inc.
- Establishment of National Institute of Biomedical Imaging
- Fluoroscopy
- Follow-up Evaluation of Radiation Oncology Patients
- Gonadal Shields
- Graduate Medical Education Funding Reform
- Hospital Risk Management Committees and Their Impact on Radiology
- Hyperthermia Guidelines
- Injection of Contrast Material and Radiopharmaceuticals
- Integrated Multidisciplinary Care of Cancer Patients
- Job Market in Radiology
- Legal Implications of Professional Courtesy
- Litigation Support Fund
- Manpower, Radiological Technology Summit Position Statement
- Manpower in Radiological Technology
- Manpower Studies
- Medical Devices: FDA Approval for Medical Devices
- Medical Dosimetrist Certification Board
- Miscellaneous Education Policies
- No Compete Clauses in Residency and Fellowship Contracts
- Nonsmoking Hospital Environment
- NRC Radiation Safety Training Requirements and Clinical Expertise in Nuclear Medicine
- Nuclear Medicine Technologist: Essentials and Guidelines of an Accredited Educational Program
- Nuclear Regulatory Commission Standards
- Opposition to a Global Tobacco Settlement
- Physics Quality Assurance Program
- Pneumoconiosis
- Practice Nonionic Contrast Agents: Equitable Pricing
- Primary Patient Access to Radiation Oncology
- Probability of Causation As a Method for Estimating Cancer Risk Associated with Radiation Exposure
- Program Director of an Accredited Educational Program in Radiological Technology: Minimum Educational Requirements
- Quality Improvement Audit Program for Radiation Oncology

- Radiation Emergencies: ACR/AMA Activity on Nonmilitary Radiation Emergencies
- Radiation Oncologist Defined
- Radiation Oncology
- Radiation Oncology Staff Privileges
- Radiation Research Program Funding
- Radiation Therapy Technologist: Essentials and Guidelines of an Accredited Educational Program
- Radiation Therapy Technologist: Title Change
- Radiographer: Essentials and Guidelines of an Accredited Educational Program
- Radiographically Identifiable Markers on Interventional Devices
- Radiological Practice and Ethics
- Radiological Technologists
- Radiological Technology Training Programs for Postgraduate Specialties
- Radiological Technology Training Programs for the Limited Radiographer
- Radiologists' Business Managers Association
- Radiology Technology Model Scholarship Agreement
- Radium: Discontinuation of Curietherapy and Disposal of Radium
- Resident and Fellowship Training Programs
- Sealed Source Application
- Simulator Capability in Radiation Therapy Facilities
- State Licensure of Medical Radiological Physicists
- State Licensure of Radiological Technologists
- Supervision of Radiological Equipment Tort Reform
- Supervision of Radiological Technologists
- Telecobalt Therapy Units
- Therapeutic Use of Unsealed Radionuclide Sources
- Uniform Terminology
- Waste Disposal Sites
- Xeromammography Equipment

American College of Rheumatology
<http://www.rheumatology.org>

Position Papers

- Access to Care
- Access to Rehabilitation for People with Rheumatic Disease
- Ambulatory Teaching
- Bone Density Measurement

- Clinical Laboratory Testing
- The Clinician-Scholar-Educator
- Complementary and Alternative Therapies for Rheumatic Disease
- Diagnostic Imaging Credentialing
- Direction of Physical and Occupational Therapy Services for Patients Under the Care of a Rheumatologist
- Fetal Tissue Research
- Guidelines for Referral of Children and Adolescents to Pediatric Rheumatologists
- Guidelines for the Practice of Arthroscopy by Rheumatologists
- Methotrexate
- New Agents for Arthritis
- Rheumatic Disease Care in Managed Health Care Systems
- The Rheumatologist as Principal Care Physician
- The Rheumatologist's Role in Providing Second Opinions for Reconstructive Orthopedic and Neurological Surgery
- The Role of Rheumatologists in Osteoporosis
- Role of Rheumatology
- Safety Guidelines for Performing Arthrocentesis
- Therapeutic Substitution
- Use of Animals in Biomedical Research

American College of Sports Medicine
<http://acsm.org/index.asp>

Position Stands

- ADA/ACSM Joint Statement: Diabetes Mellitus and Exercise
- Cardiorespiratory and Muscular Fitness, and Flexibility in Healthy Adults
- Emergency Policies at Health/Fitness Facilities
- Exercise and Fluid Replacement
- Exercise and Physical Activity for Older Adults
- Exercise and Type 2 Diabetes
- Exercise for Patients with Coronary Artery Disease
- The Female Athlete Triad
- Heat and Cold Illnesses During Distance Running
- Osteoporosis and Exercise
- Physical Activity, Physical Fitness, and Hypertension
- Proper and Improper Weight-Loss Programs
- Recommendations for Cardiovascular Screening, Staffing, and Emergency Policies of Health/Fitness Facilities

- The Recommended Quantity and Quality of Exercise for Developing and Maintaining Cardiorespiratory and Muscular Fitness and Flexibility in Healthy Adults
- The Use of Alcohol in Sports
- The Use of Anabolic-Androgenic Steroids in Sports
- The Use of Blood Doping As an Ergogenic Aid
- Weight Loss in Wrestlers

American College of Surgeons
<http://www.facs.org>

Position Statements

- Domestic Violence
- Health Care Industry Representatives in the Operating Room
- Physician Qualifications for Stereotactic Breast Biopsy: A Revised Statement
- Principles Guiding Care at the End of Life
- Recommendations for Facilities Performing Bariatric Surgery
- Statement in Response to the Clinical Alert from the National Cancer Institute
- Statement of Recommendations to Ensure Quality of Surgical Services in Managed Care Environments
- Statement of the Advisory Council for General Surgery to the Board of Regents of the American College of Surgeons
- Statement on Advance Directives by Patients: "Do Not Resuscitate" in the Operating Room
- Statement on Billing of Surgical Fees for Extracorporeal Shock Wave Lithotripsy
- Statement on Certificates of Special or Added Qualifications
- Statement on Disclosure of Commercial Interest
- Statement on Emerging Surgical Technologies and the Evaluation of Credentials
- Statement on Ethics in Patient Referrals to Ancillary Services
- Statement on Firearm Injuries
- Statement on Fundamental Characteristics of Surgical Residency Programs
- Statement on Indications for the Use of Permanently Implanted Cardiac Pacemakers
- Statement on Interprofessional Relations with Doctors of Chiropractic
- Statement on Issues to Be Considered Before New Surgical Technology Is Applied to the Care of Patients

- Statement on Laparoscopic and Thoracoscopic Procedures
- Statement on Laparoscopic Cholecystectomy
- Statement on Laser Surgery
- Statement on Managed Care and the Trauma System
- Statement on Principles Underlying Perioperative Responsibility
- Statement on Surgical Residencies and the Educational Environment
- Statement on the Physician Expert Witness
- Statement on the Surgeon and Hepatitis
- Statement on the Surgeon and HIV Infection
- Statement on the Use of Animals in Research
- Statement on the Use of Proprietary Guidelines by Managed Care Organizations
- Statement Regarding Clinical Trials
- Treatment of Patients with Calculus Disease
- Ultrasound Examinations by Surgeons

Health Policy Briefs

- Access to Health Insurance
- Access to Specialty Care
- ACS Views on Legislative, Regulatory, and Other Issues
- Ambulatory Surgical Centers
- Assistants at Surgery
- Balanced Budget Act Refinements
- Biomedical Research
- Centers of Excellence
- E&M Documentation Guidelines
- Expanding Professional Liability to Managed Care Organizations
- External Review of Health Plan Coverage and Treatment Decisions
- Fraud and Abuse
- Freedom of Choice of Physician
- Graduate Medical Education
- Managed Care Legislation
- Medical Errors and Patient Safety
- Medical Professional Liability
- Medical Records Confidentiality
- Medicare Claims Processing: Use of Commercially Developed Software
- Medicare Coverage for Clinical Trial Care
- Medicare Coverage Issues
- Medicare Fee Schedule and Related Policies

- Medicare Fee Schedule: Conversion Factor and Sustainable Growth Rate
- Medicare Fee Schedule: Practice Expenses
- Medicare Hospital Conditions of Participation
- National Practitioner Data Bank
- Office Surgery Regulation: Improving Patient Safety and Quality Care
- Patient Safety
- Postoperative Hospital Lengths of Stay
- Public Disclosure of Research Data
- Single-Use Medical Devices
- Timely Payment of Health Insurance Claims
- Trauma
- Ultrasound Guided Breast Biopsy

American Dental Association
<http://www.ada.org>

Guidelines, Positions, and Statements

- Antibiotic Prophylaxis for Dental Patients with Total Joint Replacement
- Backflow Prevention and the Dental Office
- Blood-Borne Pathogens, Infection Control, and the Practice of Dentistry
- Dental Amalgam
- Dental Mercury Hygiene Recommendations
- Dental Unit Waterlines
- Estrogenic Effects of Bisphenol A Lacking in Dental Sealants
- FDA Approval of a Laser for Hard Tissue Applications
- FDA Toothpaste Warning Labels
- Fluoride Supplementation Schedule
- Guidelines for Teaching the Comprehensive Control of Anxiety and Pain in Dentistry
- Guidelines for the Use of Conscious Sedation, Deep Sedation, and General Anesthesia for Dentistry—The Model Profession Dentists
- Infection Control Recommendations for the Dental Office and the Dental Laboratory
- Intraoral/Perioral Piercing
- New Postexposure Protocol for Occupational Exposure to Blood-Borne Diseases
- Periodontal Screening and Recording
- Phen-Fen Users

- Postexposure Evaluation and Follow-up Requirements Under OSHA's Standard for Occupational Exposure to Blood-Borne Pathogens
- Prevention of Bacterial Endocarditis
- Saliva Ejectors
- Scientists Develop Vaccine Against Tooth Decay
- Statement on Dental Anesthesia
- Statement on Water Fluoridation Efficacy and Safety
- Sugar-Free Foods and Medications
- Topical Fluorides
- Unconventional Dentistry
- The Use of Conscious Sedation, Deep Sedation, and General Anesthesia in Dentistry

American Dental Hygienists Association
<http://adha.org>

Position Statements

- Access to Care
- Educational Standards
- Managed Care
- Polishing

American Diabetes Association
<http://www.diabetes.org/homepage.jsp>

Committee Reports

- Aspirin Therapy in Diabetes
- Bedside Blood Glucose Monitoring in Hospitals
- Care of Children with Diabetes in the School and Day Care Setting
- Diabetes Mellitus and Exercise
- Diabetic Nephropathy
- Diabetic Retinopathy
- Gestational Diabetes Mellitus
- Hospital Admission Guidelines for Diabetes Mellitus
- Hypoglycemia and Employment/Licensure
- Immunization and the Prevention of Influenza and Pneumococcal Disease
- Implications of the Diabetes Control and Complications Trial
- Implications of the United Kingdom Prospective Diabetes Study
- Insulin Administration
- Management of Diabetes at Diabetes Camps

- Management of Diabetes in Correctional Institutions
- Management of Dyslipidemia in Adults with Diabetes
- Nutrition Recommendations and Principles for People with Diabetes Mellitus
- Pancreas Transplantation for Patients with Type 1 Diabetes
- Preconception Care of Women with Diabetes
- Prevention of Type 1 Diabetes Mellitus
- Preventive Foot Care in People with Diabetes
- Report of the Expert Committee on the Diagnosis and Classification of Diabetes Mellitus
- Role of Fat Replacers in Diabetes Medical Nutrition Therapy
- Screening for Type 2 Diabetes
- Smoking and Diabetes
- Standards of Medical Care for Patients with Diabetes Mellitus
- Tests of Glycemia in Diabetes
- Third-Party Reimbursement for Diabetes Care, Self-Management Education, and Supplies
- Translation of the Diabetes Nutrition Recommendations for Health Care Institutions
- Unproven Therapies

American Gastroenterological Association
<http://www.gastro.org>

Policy Statements

- AGA Wants to Know How the Proposed Practice Expense Legislation Will Impact Your Bottom Line
- Physician Fee Schedule
- Position on the Reuse of Medical Devices
- Privacy Comments for the Web
- Revisions to Payment Policies Under the Physician Fee Schedule
- Top Billed GI Codes and Impact of PE Legislation

American Geriatrics Society
<http://www.americangeriatrics.org>

Public Policy Position Statements

- Care Management Position Statement
- Comprehensive Geriatric Assessment for the Older Patient
- Conversion of Prescription Drugs to Over-the-Counter Designation
- Financing of Long-Term Care Services
- Geriatric Rehabilitation

- Home Care and Home Care Reimbursement
- Medicare
- Mental Health and the Elderly
- Physician Reimbursement Under Medicare
- Physician's Role in the Long-Term Care Facility
- Public Financing of Catastrophic Care for the Older Patient
- Research and Geriatric Medicine
- The Role of the Veterans Administration in the Care of the Elderly

Ethics Committee Position Statements

- The Care of Dying Patients
- Genetic Testing for Late-Onset Alzheimer's Disease
- Health-Screening Decisions for Older Adults
- Informed Consent for Research on Human Subjects with Dementia
- Making Treatment Decisions for Incapacitated Elderly Patients Without Advance Directives
- Physician-Assisted Suicide and Voluntary Active Euthanasia
- Rational Allocation of Medical Care
- The Responsible Conduct of Research

Health Care Systems Position Statements

- Ambulatory Geriatric Clinical Care and Services
- The Role of the Geriatrician in Managed Care

American Heart Association

<http://www.americanheart.org/presenter.jhtml?identifier=1200000>

Scientific Statements

- Aging
- Alcohol
- Aneurysm
- Angina
- Angiography
- Angioplasty
- Anticoagulants
- Antioxidants
- Arrhythmias
- Arteries
- Arteriovenous Malformation
- Aspirin
- Atherosclerosis
- Athletes
- Behavior

- Blood Pressure
- Cardiopulmonary Resuscitation
- Children
- Cholesterol
- Compliance
- Congenital Heart Defects
- Coronary Artery Bypass Graft Surgery
- Coronary Artery Calcification
- Critical Pathways
- Defibrillation
- Diabetes Mellitus
- Diet/Nutrition
- Echocardiography
- Electrocardiography
- Electron Beam
- Electrophysiology
- Emergency Cardiovascular Care
- Endocarditis
- Exercise
- Exercise Testing
- Fatty Acids
- Fibrillation
- Functional Capacity
- Genetic Testing
- Heart Attack (*see* Myocardial Infarction)
- Heart Failure
- Heart Transplant
- Heparin
- Homocysteine
- Hypertension
- Hypocholesterolemia
- Imaging
- Kawasaki Disease
- Lipids
- Mitral Valve
- Myocardial Infarction
- Nutrition
- Obesity
- Oral Anticoagulants
- Pacemakers
- Physical Activity
- Phytochemicals

- Prevention
- Protocols
- Psychotropic Drugs
- Public Access Defibrillation
- Regurgitation
- Rehabilitation
- Resuscitation
- Rheumatic Fever
- Risk Factors
- Secondary Prevention
- Sildenafil
- Smoking
- Sphygmomanometry
- Stable Angina
- Stroke
- Surgery
- Thrombosis
- Tobacco/Smoking
- Tomography, Electron Beam Computed
- Trans-Fatty Acids
- Transient Ischemic Attack
- "Utstein Style" Reporting Guidelines
- Vascular Heart Disease
- Vascular Medicine
- Weight Management
- Women

American Hospital Association
<http://www.hospitalconnect.com/hospitalconnect/index.jsp>

Policy Briefs
- Implications of President Clinton's Plan to Modernize the Traditional Fee-for-Service Managed Care/Consumer Protection Legislation
- Medicare Program
- President Clinton's Plan to Reform Medicare
- Prompt Payment of Providers

Position Statements
- AHA Position on HHS' Denial of Medicare Losses in Nonprofit M&As
- Hospital Disaster Plans in New York and Washington, DC

- MedPAC's GME Report
- Principles and Guidelines for Changes in Hospital Ownership
- Principles for Confidentiality of Health Information
- Statement on Hospital Compliance Programs

American Industrial Hygiene Association
<http://www.aiha.org>

Position Statements
- AIHA Position on 29 CFR Part 1910, Ergonomics Program; Proposed Rule
- AIHA's View of Occupational Health and Safety on a National and Global Scale
- Environmental Lead
- Ergonomics
- Extremely Low Frequency and Magnetic Fields
- National Environmental Laboratory Accreditation
- Occupational M. Tuberculosis
- OHS Performance Criteria in Contracting and Procurement
- Permissible Exposure Limits
- Pollution Prevention and Toxic Use Reduction
- Position on Sweatshops in the Global Economy
- Position Statement on Prevention of Workplace Violence
- Recording Occupational Hearing Loss
- Risk Assessment and Risk Management
- Third-Party Workplace Reviews
- Total Human Exposure
- Workplace Rights Position Paper

White Papers
- AIHA's View of Occupational Health and Safety on a National and Global Scale
- Generic Exposure Assessment Standard
- Global Hazard Communication
- Occupational M. Tuberculosis
- OHS Performance Criteria in Contracting and Procurement
- Permissible Exposure Limits
- Prevention of Workplace Violence
- Risk Assessment and Risk Management
- Sweatshops in the Global Economy
- Total Human Exposure
- Workplace Rights

American Institute of Ultrasound in Medicine

<http://aium.org>

Official Statements and Reports

- AIUM's Role in the Legislative Arena
- Clinical Safety
- Conclusions Regarding Epidemiology
- Conclusions Regarding Gas Bodies
- Conclusions Regarding Heat
- Conclusions Regarding Tissue Models and Equipment Survey
- Definition of a Final Report
- Diagnostic Spinal Ultrasound
- Improving Delivery and Quality of Ultrasound Services
- Interpretation of Ultrasound Examinations
- In Vitro Biological Effects
- Limited Obstetrical Ultrasound
- Mammalian In Vivo Ultrasonic Biological Effects
- Manufacturers Are Encouraged to Publish Acoustic Parameters
- Providing Images to Patients
- Prudent Use
- Recommendations for Cleaning Transabdominal Transducers
- Recommendations for Inclusion on Written Reports
- Reimbursable Obstetrical Ultrasound
- Safety in Training and Research
- Third Party Accreditation Reporting Packages
- 3D Technology
- Training Guidelines for Physicians Who Evaluate and Interpret Diagnostic Ultrasound Examinations

American Liver Foundation

<http://www.liverfoundation.org>

Position Statements

- Acetaminophen Use and Liver Injury
- Hepatitis B Vaccination

American Managed Behavioral Healthcare Association

<http://www.ambha.org>

Public Policy Statements

- AMBHA-ASAM Joint Statement on Practice Guidelines
- Any Willing Provider
- Bill of Rights for Consumers Accessing Behavioral Health Services

- Clinically Appropriate Access to Medical Records
- Medicaid's IMD Prohibition
- Parity in Benefit Coverage: A Joint AMBHA-ASAM Statement
- Parity in Benefit Design
- Provider-Sponsored Organizations
- Statement of Confidentiality
- Statement on Co-occurring Disorders

American Medical Students Association
<http://www.amsa.org>

Health Policy Issues

- Fact Sheet on the Corps
- Fact Sheet on the Patients' Bill of Rights
- Funding of Graduate Medical Education
- Gay/Lesbian Rights
- GME Funding and the "All-Payer" Act Primer
- Hate Crimes Fact Sheet
- H.R. 2391, the National Center for Research on Domestic Health Disparities Act
- H.R. 3250, the Health Care Fairness Act
- H.R. 4483, the Women's Health Office Act of 2000
- Letter and Fact Sheet on GME Funding
- Letter on GME Funding from AMSA to the Senate Finance Committee
- Medical Record Privacy
- Minority Health Issues
- National Health Service Corps
- Patents on Genetic Materials
- Patients' Bill of Rights
- Pharmaceutical Industry
- Physician Collective Bargaining
- Prescription Drug Primer
- Prescription Drugs
- A Primer for Medical Students
- A Primer on Gene Patents
- A Primer on Women and Tobacco: The Leading American Epidemic
- Primer on Physician Unionization and the "Campbell Bill"
- Primer on the Corps
- Resident Work Hours
- Tobacco

- Tobacco Control Action Packet
- Universal Health Care
- Women's Health Issues

American Medical Women's Association
<http://www.amwa-doc.org>

Position Papers

- Abuse in Medical Education and Training Programs
- Advance Directives
- Breast Cancer Detection
- Breast Cancer Diagnosis
- Breast Cancer Prevention
- Breast Cancer Screening
- Breast Cancer Treatment
- Care of the Dependent Elderly
- Cerebrovascular Disease in Women
- Dependent Care
- Domestic Violence
- Emergency Contraception
- Ethics on Managed Care
- Gender Discrimination and Sexual Harassment
- Genetic Testing for Breast and Ovarian Cancer Susceptibility
- Health Care Reform
- Health Care Reform and Women's Health
- Lesbian Health Issues
- Maternity Leave
- Medicaid Program Reform
- Minority Women's Health
- Physician-Assisted Suicide
- Pregnancy During Schooling, Training, and Early Practice Years
- Principles of Ethical Conduct
- Reproductive Health
- Tobacco Control and Prevention
- Women and Coronary Heart Disease

American Nephrology Nurses Association
<http://annanurse.org>

Position Statements

- Advanced Practice in Nephrology Nursing
- Apolitical Educational Programs

- Autonomy of the Nephrology Nursing Certification Commission
- Certification in Nephrology Nursing
- Collaboration Between Nephrologists and Advanced Practice Nurses
- Concerns Regarding Inclusion of End-Stage Renal Disease Patients in Managed Care Plans
- Daily Hemodialysis/Nocturnal Hemodialysis
- Delegation of Nursing Care Activities
- Financial Incentives for Organ Donation
- The Impact of the National Nursing Shortage on Quality Nephrology Nursing Care
- Minimum Preparation for Entry into Nursing Practice
- Solicitation or Offering of Human Organs and Tissues for Transplantation for Financial Gain
- Unlicensed Assistive Personnel in Dialysis Therapy
- Unlicensed Personnel in Dialysis
- Vascular Access for Dialysis

American Neurotology Society
<http://www.otology-neurotology.org/ANS/ans-main.html>

Policy Statements

- Components of the Neurotologic Examination
- Facial Nerve Monitoring

Joint Policy Statements: American Neurotologic Society and American Otologic Society

- Cochlear Implants
- Dynamic Posturography and Vestibular Testing
- Evaluation Prior to Hearing Aid Fitting
- Facial Nerve Monitoring
- Hearing Aids
- Hearing Impairment
- Implantable Hearing Devices
- Infant Hearing
- Institution-Based Audiology Facilities
- Medical Role in Cerumen Removal

American Orthopaedic Foot and Ankle Society
<http://aofas.org>

Position Statements

- Endoscopic and Open Heel Surgery

- Hospital and Medical Organization Credentialing
- Preventing Lawn Mower Injuries
- The Provision of Quality Foot and Ankle Care in the United States
- The Role of Breakaway Bases in Preventing Recreational Baseball and Softball Injuries
- Women's Shoes and Foot Problems

American Pain Society
<http://www.ampainsoc.org>

Position Statements

- Health Care Policy Statement
- Pain Assessment and Treatment in the Managed Care Environment
- Pain: The Fifth Vital Sign
- Pediatric Chronic Pain
- Treatment of Pain at the End of Life
- The Use of Opioids for the Treatment of Chronic Pain

American Pharmacists Association
<http://www.aphanet.org>

Policy Statements

- Collective Bargaining/Unionization
- Employer/Employee Communications
- Employment Standards
- Unionization of Pharmacists: State Participation in Employer/Employee Relations
- Working Conditions on Public Safety

American Physical Therapy Association
<http://apta.org>

Policies and Positions

- Chapter Responsibility Concerning Medicaid
- Clinical Continuing Education for Individuals Other Than Physical Therapists
- Education Program Development and Expansion in Physical Therapy
- Entry Point into Health Care
- Goals That Represent the 2003 Priorities of the American Physical Therapy Association
- Insurance Benefits for Physical Therapy Services
- Integrity in Serving the Association

- Licensure: Qualified Exemption
- Physical Education Advocacy
- Physical Therapist Assistants
- Physical Therapist Ownership and Operation of Physical Therapy Services
- Physical Therapy Association
- Physical Therapy for Older Adults
- Primary Care and the Role of the Physical Therapist
- Professional Education and Designation of the Physical Therapist
- Professional Practice Relationships
- Recommendations for Nomination for National Office
- Transition DPT: Accessibility to Degree Programs

American Psychiatric Association
<http://www.psych.org>

Issue Briefs

- Addressing the Mental Health Needs of America's Children
- APA Principles—Restructured Medicaid Program
- APA Seclusion and Restraint Resource Guide
- APA's 12 Principles of National Health Care Reform
- Confidentiality Fact Sheet
- Current Issue Brief—Seclusion and Restraint
- Current Issue Brief—VA Prescribing Authority
- Department of Defense Psychopharmacology Demonstration Project Fact Sheet
- Fact Sheet/Chart on Senator James Jeffords' Proposed Confidentiality Legislation
- Graduate Medical Education Policy for Psychiatry Fact Sheet
- Insurance Coverage Parity for Mental Illness Treatment Fact Sheet
- Key Children's Mental Health Legislation in the 107th Congress
- Medical Records Privacy
- Medicare and Managed Care Fact Sheet
- Medicare and Mental Illness Treatment Fact Sheet
- Medicare Discrimination Against Mental Illness Treatment
- Medicare Physician Payment Update
- Medicare Prescription Drug Coverage
- Medicare Private Contracting
- Medicare Regulatory Fairness
- Mental Health Parity—Its Time Has Come
- New Federal Investments in Psychiatric Research
- Nonphysician Mental Health Practitioners Fact Sheet

- Patient Protection
- Principles for Medical Record Privacy Legislation
- Research and Services for Mental Illnesses Fact Sheet
- Resource-Based Practice Expenses Under Medicare's RBRVS Fact Sheet
- Resource-Based Relative Value Scale Medicare Fee Schedule Fact Sheet
- Scope of Practice: Psychologist Prescribing Legislation
- Toward the Millennium: Universal Access to Psychiatric Care
- Veterans Affairs Issues in Psychiatric Research

American Psychiatric Nurses Association
<http://apna.org>

Position Papers
- Determining Staffing Needs of Inpatient Psychiatric Units
- Mandatory Outpatient Treatment
- Prescriptive Authority for Advanced Practice Psychiatric Nurses
- Professional Titling and Credentialing
- Psychiatric–Mental Health Nurse Roles Outcomes Evaluation and Management Collaboration
- Psychiatric–Mental Health Nursing Practice
- Roles of Psychiatric–Mental Health Nurses in Managed Care
- Seclusion and Restraint Standards of Practice
- Use of Seclusion and Restraint

American Public Health Association
<http://apha.org>

Policy Statements
- Abortion
- Acid rain
- Adolescent Health
- Aedes aegypti
- Affirmative Action
- Africa
- AIDS
- Ambulatory Care
- Apartheid
- Arctic
- Armed forces
- Asbestos

- Behavioral Sciences
- Benzene
- Bicycles
- Birth Centers
- Birth Certificates
- Birth Defects
- Birth Registration
- Bleach
- Blood
- Boxing
- Boycott
- Cancer
- Capital Punishment
- Catastrophic Illness
- Censorship
- Cesarean Section
- Chemicals
- Child Health and Development
- Chiropractic
- Chronic Illness
- Cigarettes
- Citizen Action Groups
- Civil Rights
- Community Health Programs
- Compensation
- Consumerism
- Contact Lenses
- Contraceptives
- Coronary Heart Disease
- Correctional Facilities
- Cost Containment
- Counseling
- Crime
- Cuba
- Cutbacks
- Day Care
- Deinstitutionalization
- Diabetes
- Diagnostic Services
- Diphtheria Tetanus Pertussis
- Disabled Persons
- Disasters

- Disease Reporting
- District of Columbia
- Divestment
- Domestic Animals
- Drinking Age
- Driver Safety
- Drug Coding
- Education
- El Salvador
- Emergency Medical Services
- Employment
- Endoscopes
- Energy
- English Only
- Environment
- Epilepsy
- Equal Rights Amendment
- Ethics
- Ethiopia
- Ethylene Dibromide
- Ethylene Oxide
- Excise Taxes
- Family Health
- Family Planning
- Famine
- Federal Appropriations
- Federal Health Services
- Fertility Regulation
- Food Stamps
- Formaldehyde
- Fraud
- Freedom of Information
- Future of Public Health
- Genetics
- Geriatric Health
- Grants-in-Aid
- Grenada
- Haiti
- Handicapped Persons
- Hazards
- Health Care Fraud
- Health Education

- Health Insurance
- Health Maintenance Organizations
- Health Planning and Administration
- Health Records
- Hepatitis
- Hill-Burton Program
- Hispanics
- HIV
- Homeless
- Homosexuality
- Hospice
- Hospitals
- Housing
- Human Rights
- Immigrants
- Immunization
- Indians
- Indochina
- Infectious Disease
- Injury Control
- International Health
- Jail/Prisons
- Journals and Publications
- Kidney Dialysis
- Korea
- Laboratory
- Land Use
- Language
- Laws
- Lead Poisoning
- Local Health Services
- Long-Term Care
- Malaria
- Malpractice
- Managed Care
- Measles
- Medicaid
- Medical Care
- Medical Care Costs
- Medical Devices
- Mental Health
- Mental Retardation

- Midwives
- Migrant Health
- Military
- Milk
- Minorities
- Mopeds
- Mortality
- Mosquitoes
- Motor Vehicles
- Multiphasic Screening
- Narcotics
- National Driver Register
- National Health Policy
- Native Americans
- Naturopathy
- Neighborhood Health Centers
- Nestle
- Nicaragua
- Nuclear Testing
- Nutrition
- Nutrition Education
- Occupational Health and Safety
- Oleomargarine
- Oral Health
- Ozone
- Paperwork Reduction Act
- Parental Notification
- Patient Dumping
- Patient's Rights
- Peace Corps
- Persian Gulf War
- Personnel
- Pets
- Pharmaceuticals
- Physical Fitness
- Pit And Fissure Sealants
- Podiatric Health
- Politics
- Pollution
- Populations/Family Planning
- Poverty
- Pregnancy

- Prevention
- Privacy
- Professional Education and Training
- Professionalism
- Public Interest Groups
- Quality Assurance
- Rabies
- Racism
- Radiological Health
- Radon
- Reimbursement
- Reproductive Health
- Research
- Right-to-Know
- Rural Health
- Sanitation
- School Health
- Screening
- Security
- Sexually Transmitted Diseases
- Sickle Cell
- Smallpox
- Smokeless Tobacco
- Smoking
- Social Sciences
- South Africa
- State Health Services
- Statistics
- Strategic Defense Initiative
- Substance Abuse
- Sudden Infant Death Syndrome
- Sulfur Dioxide
- Surgery
- Taxation
- Television
- Tissue Transplants
- Tobacco
- Trade
- Trichinosis
- Tuberculosis
- Unemployment

- Urban Health
- Uruguay
- Veterans Administration
- Veterinary Public Health
- Video Display Terminals
- Vietnam War
- Violence
- Vision Care
- Voters
- Warning Labels
- Water
- Welfare
- White House
- WIC
- Women's Health
- Workers' Compensation
- World Health Organization
- Yellow Fever

American Society for Clinical Laboratory Science
<http://www.ascls.org>

Position Statements

- Health Care Reform
- Independent Practice
- Leukoreduced Blood Products
- Managed Care
- Medical Errors and Patient Safety
- Point of Care

American Society for Dermatologic Surgery
<http://www.asds-net.org>

Policy and Issues

- Definition of the Practice of Medicine
- Does the Location of the Surgery or the Specialty of the Physician Affect Malpractice Claims in Liposuction?
- Practice of Medicine and Use of Nonphysician Office Personnel
- Use of Lasers, Intense Pulsed Light, Radio Frequency, and Medical Microwave Devices

American Society for Gastrointestinal Endoscopy
<http://asge.org>

Health Policy

- Hospital Outpatient Department Prospective Payment System

American Society for Health System Pharmacists
<http://www.ashp.org>

Issue Papers

- Any Willing Provider/Freedom of Choice
- Collaborative Drug Therapy Management
- Confidentiality of Patient Medical Records
- The Delicate Balance Between Internet Pharmacy and Patient Safety
- Drug Samples
- The Expanding Role of the Pharmacist and the Reimbursement Dilemma
- FDA Reform
- Formulary Systems and National/State Formularies
- Graduate Medical Education and Funding for Pharmacy Residencies
- Medicare Prescription Drug Coverage and Pharmacists' Professional Patient Care Services
- The Misnamed "Pain Relief Promotion Act"
- Patient Safety and Medical Errors
- Pharmaceutical Price Discounts
- Unlabeled Uses of Medications/Dissemination of Information/Reimbursement by Third Parties

Policy Positions

- Abbreviated New Drug Applications; Generic Drugs
- Access to Pharmacists
- Accreditation; Residencies
- Administration Devices; Pharmacist's Role
- Administration of Medications; Pharmacist's Role
- Administration Systems; Manufacturer's Role
- Administrators
- Adulteration, *see* Counterfeit Drugs
- Adverse Drug Reaction; Reporting
- Advertising; Direct-to-Consumer
- Affiliated Chapters, *see* State Chapters
- AHA, *see* American Hospital Association

- AIDS, *see* Human Immunodeficiency Virus
- Alcohol Abuse
- Alcoholics Anonymous; Impaired Pharmacists
- Alternative Delivery Sites, *see* Nontraditional Practice Settings
- Ambulatory Care
- American Association of Colleges of Pharmacy; Hospital Practice Sites
- American College of Hospital Administrators; Materials Management
- American Council on Pharmaceutical Education
- American Hospital Association
- American Hospital Formulary Service; Development
- American Pharmaceutical Association
- Annual Meeting; Registration Fees
- Apothecary System; Elimination
- Appearance; Generic Drugs
- Appointments; Qualifications
- Apportionment
- Assisted Suicide
- Blood Products Management
- Blue Cross/Blue Shield; Reimbursement
- Bulk Resale of Drugs; Legislation
- Business Leaders; Patient Care Policy Responsibilities
- Capital Punishment
- Careers; Counseling
- Chemical Dependence
- Clerkships
- Clinical Drug Research
- Clinical Pharmacy Services
- Codes
- Collaborative Drug Therapy
- Colleges of Pharmacy
- Competency; Education, Continuing
- Complementary and Alternative Substances
- Compounding versus Manufacturing
- Computers
- Confidentiality of Patient Health Care Information
- Confidentiality; Patient Information
- Conscientious Objection
- Consulting Firms, External; Communication with
- Consumer Education
- Contents on Package Labels

- Continuing Education
- Control
- Controlled Substances
- Cost Containment, Pharmacy Services
- Cost-effectiveness
- Council on Educational Affairs; Responsibilities
- Council on Therapeutics
- Counterfeit Drugs; Legislation
- Crime; Pharmacy; Law Enforcement
- Curriculum; Education, Undergraduate
- Data Collection
- Degrees
- Delegate Representation
- Delegates; Registration Fees
- Designer Drugs
- Dietary Supplements
- Directors of Pharmacy
- Direct-to-Consumer Advertising
- Disease Management Plans
- Dispensing; Pharmacists Without Prescription
- Doctor of Pharmacy Degree; Entry-Level
- Dosage Forms
- Downsizing the Pharmacy Department
- Drug Abuse, *see* Substance Abuse
- Drug Control
- Drug Costs
- Drug Delivery Systems
- Drug Distribution
- Drug Enforcement Administration
- Drug Information (Medication Information)
- Drug Price Competition Act; Generic Drugs
- Drug Therapy
- Dues Rate
- Dying Patients
- Economics, *see* Reimbursement, Cost Containment, Cost-effectiveness
- Education
- Education, Medical; Funding
- Education, Postgraduate
- Education, Undergraduate
- Electronic Communication of Medical Information
- Electronic Entry; Medication Orders, Prescriptions

- Electronic Information Systems
- Emergency Preparedness
- Employment
- Ethics
- Expanded Services, *see* Nontraditional Practice Settings
- Expiration Dates; Pharmaceutical Products
- FDA, *see* Food and Drug Administration
- Financial Management
- Financial Programs
- Financing, *see* Reimbursement
- Food and Drug Administration
- Formulary System
- Generic Drug Products
- Geriatrics; Clinical Trials
- Goals; Long-Range Planning
- Governing Process
- Graduate Medical Education Funding
- Health Care Financing, *see* Reimbursement
- Health Care Reform
- Health Risks; Alcohol and Other Substances
- Home Care
- Home Intravenous Therapy; Reimbursement
- Hospital Financial Management Association; Reimbursement
- Human Immunodeficiency Virus
- Identification
- Immunization; Pharmacist's Role
- Impaired Pharmacists
- Indications, New; FDA Approval
- Industry, *see* Pharmaceutical Manufacturers
- Infection Control, Pharmacist's Role in
- Information
- Informed Consent; Clinical Trials
- Institutional Review Boards
- International System of Units (SI Units); Labeling
- Internships; Education, Undergraduate
- Investigational Drug
- Investigational Review Boards; Liaisons
- Jails, *see* Correctional Facilities
- Joint Commission on Accreditation of Health Care Organizations
- Labeling; Medication, Drug Products
- Law Enforcement; Pharmacy Crime
- Leadership

- Long-Range Planning; Goals
- Managed-Care Settings; Pharmacy Practice in
- Managers; Pharmacy
- Manpower; Data Collection
- Marketing; Nontraditional Practice Settings
- Materials Management
- Medication Administration
- Medication Errors
- Medication Misadventures
- Medication Orders; Prescriptions
- Medication-Use Policy Development, *see* Formulary System
- Medication-Use Process; Performance Improvement
- Mentors; Pharmacy Managers
- Midyear Clinical Meeting
- Misbranding, *see* Counterfeit Drugs
- Models; Clinical Trials
- Multidisciplinary Action Plans
- National Association of Boards of Pharmacy
- National Drug Code
- Needle and Syringe Exchange
- Nondiscriminatory Pharmaceutical Care
- Nontraditional Practice Settings
- Nutritional Support Pharmacy; Recognition As a Specialty
- Organ Transplantation, *see* Transplantation
- Outcome Indicators, *see* Patient Outcomes
- Outpatient Services, *see* Ambulatory Care
- Packaging
- Pain Management
- Patient Assistance
- Patient Care
- Patient-Focused Care
- Patient Information, *see* Information
- Patient Outcomes
- Patients; Right to Choose
- Payment Policies; Government
- Pediatric
- Performance Improvement; Medication-Use Process
- Pharmaceutical Care
- Pharmaceutical Manufacturers
- Pharmaceutical Research in Organized Health Care Settings
- Pharmacist Decision Making in Assisted Suicide
- Pharmacist Dispensing Without a Prescription

- Pharmacist in Patient-Focused Care; Approval
- Pharmacist's Responsibility for Distribution and Control of Drugs
- Pharmacist's Role in Clinical Pharmacokinetic Monitoring
- Pharmacist's Role in Infection Control
- Pharmacist's Role in Primary Care
- Pharmacist's Role in Substance Abuse Prevention, Education, and Assistance
- Pharmacist's Role with Respect to Drug Delivery Systems and Administration Devices
- Pharmacokinetic Monitoring, Pharmacist's Role in
- Pharmacy and Therapeutics Committee, *see* Formulary System
- Pharmacy, Organized Health Care Settings; Promoting Image of
- Pharmacy Technicians
- Practice Settings
- Practice Sites for Undergraduates; Health Systems
- Preceptors
- Prescriptions, *see* Medication Orders
- Preventive Care; Role for Pharmacists
- Prices; Drug Product
- Primary Care; Role for Pharmacists
- Productivity Monitoring and Reporting
- Professional Competency, *see* Competency
- Professional Image, *see* Public Relations
- Proxy/Absentee Ballots
- Psychopharmacy; Recognition As a Specialty
- Publications
- Public Relations
- Purchasing (Procurement)
- Quality of Clinical Services
- Records; Drug Enforcement Administration
- Recruitment Materials
- Recycling; Pharmaceutical Waste
- Registration Fees; Delegates
- Regulations
- Reimbursement
- Research
- Residencies
- Resizing the Pharmacy Department
- Right to Choose; Patients
- Risk Management; Medication Errors
- Robbery, *see* Crime
- Route of Administration; FDA Approval

- Sales; Bulk Resale of Drugs
- Samples, *see* Drug Samples
- Single-Unit Packaging; Problems
- SI Units, *see* International System of Units
- Smoking
- Software
- Specialties; Pharmacy Practice
- Staff Development; Director of Pharmacy Support; ASHP Assistance
- State Chapters
- Student Membership Dues
- Substance Abuse
- Support for Interdisciplinary Patient Care Training
- Supportive Personnel, *see* Technicians
- Surveys, *see* Data Collection
- Tamper-Evident Packaging on Topical Products
- Technicians, *see* Pharmacy Technicians
- Teleconferences
- Telepharmacy
- Terrorism; Chemical and Biological
- Therapeutic Interchange
- Therapeutics, Council on; Proposed Creation of
- Therapeutic Substitution
- Third-Party Compensation, *see* Reimbursement
- Third-Party Compensation for Clinical Services by Pharmacists
- Tobacco; Use and Distribution in Pharmacies
- Transplantation; Reimbursement for Related Drugs and Services
- Undergraduate Education, *see* Education, Undergraduate
- Unit Dose Drug Distribution
- Unlabeled Drug Use; Reimbursement
- Use of Medications for Unlabeled Uses
- Vaccines; Availability
- Waste; Pharmaceutical; Recycling
- Wholesalers; Electronic Data Interchange
- Workload Monitoring and Reporting

American Society for Interventional and Therapeutic Neuroradiology
<http://asitn.org>

Position Statement

- Interventional Stroke Therapy

American Society for Investigative Pathology
<http://asip.org>

Position Statement

- Human Tissues in Genetic Research

American Society for Microbiology
<http://www.asm.org>

Position Statements

- Apple Juice
- Biomedical Research
- Genetically Modified Organisms
- Institute of Medicine's Study on Medicare Payment Methodology for Clinical Laboratory Services
- Scientific Principles to Guide Biological Weapons Verification, 1993
- Use of Antibiotic-Resistant Marker Genes in Transgenic Plants

American Society for Nutritional Sciences
<http://www.nutrition.org>

Position Statements

- Food Labeling
- Food Programs
- Objections to "Seal of Approval" Programs
- Resolution on Fluoridation of Drinking Water
- Vitamin and Mineral Supplements

American Society for Pharmacology and Experimental Therapeutics
<http://aspet.org>

Position Statements

- Herbal Medicine and Pharmacological Research
- Stem Cell Research

American Society for Reproductive Medicine
<http://asrm.org>

Position Statements

- Definition of "Experimental"
- Definition of "Infertility"
- Electroejaculation
- Intracytoplasmic Sperm Injection
- Oral Contraceptives and Thromboembolic Events

American Society for Surgery of the Hand
<http://www.assh.org>

Policy Statement

- Hand Transplantation

American Society of Addiction Medicine
<http://asam.org>

Public Policy

- Addiction Medicine: Basic Concepts
- Addictive Diseases
- Children and Addiction
- Commercial Products and Advertising
- Diagnosis
- Drugs: Alcohol
- Drugs: Marijuana
- Drugs: Nicotine
- Drugs: Opiates
- Economic Aspects of Addiction and Treatment
- Ethics and Confidentiality
- Forensics and Criminal Justice Policy
- HIV/AIDS and Addiction
- Medical Aspects of Substance Use and Addiction
- Motor Vehicles and Highway Safety
- National Drug Policy
- Occupational Aspects of Substance Use, Addiction, and Treatment
- Practice of Addiction Medicine
- Prescription Drugs
- Prevention
- Professional Impairment
- Psychiatric Aspects of Substance Use and Addiction
- Public Health
- Recovery
- Research and Evaluation
- Screening
- Substance Use
- Treatment of Addictive Disorders
- Women and Addiction

American Society of Breast Surgeons
<http://www.breastsurgeons.org>

Official Statements
- Ablative and Percutaneous Treatment of Breast Cancer
- Image-Guided Percutaneous Biopsy of Palpable Breast Lesions

American Society of Cataract and Refractive Surgery
<http://ascrs.org>

Position Statement
- Coalition for Fair Medicare Payment

American Society of Clinical Oncology
<http://asco.org/ac/1,1003,_12-002138,00.asp>

Policy Issues
- CAM Therapies
- Clinical Trials
- Genetic Testing
- Medical Records Privacy
- Palliative Care
- Quality Cancer Care
- Stem Cell Research
- Tobacco Control

American Society of Consultant Pharmacists
<http://www.ascp.com>

Policy Statements
- Automation in Pharmacy
- Capitation
- Collaborative Practice
- Competence, Continuing, for Pharmacists
- Compliance with Fraud and Abuse Laws
- Controlled Drugs in Nursing Facilities
- Counseling Geriatric Patients
- Drug and Related Research in the Elderly
- Drug Pricing
- Formularies in Nursing Facilities
- Geriatrics, Inclusion in the Pharmacy School Curriculum
- Immunization
- Inappropriate Business Practices

- Infection Control, Role of the Consultant Pharmacist in Long-Term Care Facilities
- Initial Doses of Medications for Nursing Facility Residents
- Interdisciplinary Team
- Mandatory Tablet Splitting for Cost Containment
- Medicare Prescription Benefit
- Medication Errors, Preventing, in Pharmacies and Long-Term Care Facilities
- Narrow Therapeutic Index Drugs
- Patient Advocacy, Role of the Consultant Pharmacist in
- Payment for Pharmaceutical Care
- Pharmaceutical Care
- Pharmacy Technicians in Long-Term Care Pharmacy
- Prescription Orders, Including Therapeutic Purpose
- Prescriptive Authority for Pharmacists
- Resident Assessment and Care Planning, Role of the Consultant Pharmacist
- Return and Reuse of Medications in Long-Term Care Facilities
- Separation of Providers and Consultants

American Society of Cytopathology
<http://www.cytopathology.org>

Position Statements

- Guidelines for Review of Gynecologic Cytology Samples I: The Context of Litigation and Potential Litigation
- Proposed Guidelines for Primary Screening Instruments for Gynecologic Cytology
- A Proposed Methodology for Evaluating Secondary Screening Instruments for Gynecologic Cytology
- Technical Devices for Innovation in Cervical Cytology Screening

American Society of Electroneurodiagnostic Technologists
<http://aset.org/home>

Position Statements

- Electroneurodiagnostic Technologists in the Operating Room
- Invasive Electrode Techniques
- Licensure for Electroneurodiagnostic Technologists
- Minimal Educational Requirements for Performing Electroneurodiagnostic Procedures
- Multicompetency and Cross Training

- National Competencies for Performing an Electroencephalogram
- National Competencies for Performing Evoked Potential Studies
- Simultaneous Intraoperative Monitoring
- Statement of Professional Ethics
- Technologists Administering Sedation
- Technologists Performing Apnea Studies
- Utilization of Professional Credentials

American Society of General Surgeons
<http://www.theasgs.org>

Position Statements

- Ambulatory Surgical Centers
- Image-Guided Breast Biopsies
- Patients' Rights: Statements of Principles
- Scope of Practice and Credentialing
- The Specialty of General Surgery and the Definition of a General Surgeon
- Surgeons As Assistants in Surgery

American Society of Gene Therapy
<http://asgt.org>

Position Statements

- Financial Conflict of Interest in Clinical Research
- Reporting of Patient Adverse Events in Gene Therapy Trials

American Society of Hematology
<http://www.hematology.org>

Policy Statement

- Adult and Embryonic Stem Cell Research

American Society of Human Genetics
<http://www.ashg.org/genetics/ashg/ashgmenu.htm>

Policy Statements

- Clinical Genetics and Freedom of Choice
- Cystic Fibrosis Carrier Screening
- DNA Banking and DNA Analysis: Points to Consider
- Eugenics and the Misuse of Genetic Information to Restrict Reproductive Freedom
- Family History and Privacy Advisory

- Gene Therapy
- Genetic Testing and Insurance
- Genetic Testing for Breast and Ovarian Cancer Predisposition
- Genetic Testing in Adoption
- Informed Consent for Genetic Research
- Mapping/Sequencing the Human Genome
- Maternal Serum Alpha-Fetoprotein Screening Programs and Quality Control for Laboratories
- Patenting of Expressed Sequence Tags
- Points to Consider: Ethical, Legal, and Psychosocial Implications of Genetic Testing in Children and Adolescents
- Professional Disclosure of Familial Genetic Information
- Recent Developments in Human Behavioral Genetics
- Sharing Research Data
- Stem Cell Research
- Tandem Mass Spectrometry in Newborn Screening
- Use of Apolipoprotein E Testing for Alzheimer's Disease

American Society of Internal Medicine (an affiliate of ACP)
<http://www.acponline.org/>

Position Statements

- Access to Care
- Antitrust
- Bioterrorism
- Fraud and Abuse
- Graduate Medical Education
- Liability
- Managed Care
- Medicare Issues
- Patient Safety/IOM Report
- Physician Payment, Coding, and Billing
- Prescription Drug Benefit
- Privacy
- Tobacco

American Society of Interventional and Therapeutic Neuroradiology
<http://asitn.org>

Position Statement

- Emergency Interventional Stroke Therapy

American Society of Nuclear Cardiology
<http://asnc.org>

Policy/Position Statements

- Cardiac Radionuclide Imaging—Guidelines for Clinical Use
- Clinical Application of Radionuclide Angiography
- Clinical Relevance of a Normal Myocardial Perfusion Scintigraphic Study
- Credentials Recommended for Cardiologists Seeking Hospital Privileges to Perform Nuclear Cardiology Procedures
- Design and Implementation of a Nuclear Cardiology Testing Facility in a Private-Practice Cardiology Office Setting
- ECG Gating of Myocardial Perfusion SPECT Scintigrams
- Imaging Guidelines for Nuclear Cardiology Procedures, Part I and II
- Mobile and Remote-Site Provision of Nuclear Cardiology Imaging Services
- Nonperfusion Applications in Nuclear Cardiology
- Training in Nuclear Cardiology—ACC/ASNC Recommendations
- Wintergreen Panel Summaries

American Society of Perianesthesia Nurses
<http://aspan.org>

Position Statements

- Air Safety in the Perianesthesia Environment
- Fast Tracking
- ICU Overflow Patients
- Minimum Staffing in Phase I PACU
- Nursing Shortage
- On Call/Work Schedule
- Pain Management
- Perianesthesia Advanced Practice Nursing
- The Perianesthesia Patient with a Do-Not-Resuscitate Advance Directive
- Registered Nurse Utilization of Unlicensed Assistive Personnel

American Society of Plastic Surgeons
<http://www.plasticsurgery.org>

Position Papers

- Abdominoplasty
- Blepharoplasty and Eyelid Reconstruction
- Breast Reconstruction

- Carpal Tunnel Syndrome
- Cleft Lip and Palate Surgery
- Cutaneous Laser Surgery
- Ear Deformity: Prominent Ears
- Endoscopic Surgery—Qualifications to Perform
- Gynecomastia
- Health Care for the Reconstruction of Abnormal Appearance
- Nasal Surgery
- Orthognathic Surgery
- Prior Authorization/Predetermination
- Prophylactic Mastectomy
- Reoperation/Breast Implants
- Scar Revision
- Skin Lesions
- Treatment of Skin Redundancy Following Massive Weight Loss

American Society of Radiologic Technologists
<https://www.asrt.org>

Position Statements
- Health Care Delivery Systems and Health Care Policy
- Support of the American Hospital Association's Patient's Bill of Rights

Public Health Statements
- Advanced Professional Career Levels
- Brachytherapy Remote Afterloading Equipment
- Breast Palpation by Radiologic Technologists
- Certification of Personnel Practicing in the Radiologic Sciences
- Conjoint Evaluation of Educational Programs
- Definition of Multicredentialed Radiologic Technologist
- Degree Requirements for Radiologic Science Program Directors and Faculty
- Diagnostic Radiographic Imaging
- Drug Administration by Radiologic Technologists
- Educational Level for Advanced Specialties
- Fluoroscopic Guidance for Contrast Studies of the Gastrointestinal System
- Fluoroscopy by Radiologic Technologists
- HIV and Hepatitis Testing for Health Care Workers
- Hyperthermia

- Identification of Registered Radiologic Technologists in the Workplace
- Institutional Licensure of Radiologic Technologists
- International System of Units
- Level of Education for the Radiologic Science Profession
- Licensure and Certification Issues
- Limited Radiography
- Multiskilled Radiologic Technologists
- Nondiscrimination in the Practice of the Radiologic Sciences
- Operation of Simulation and Radiation Therapy Treatment Units
- Placement of Intravascular Closure Devices
- Professional Advancement in the Radiologic Sciences
- Professional Continuing Education
- Professional Issues for Clinical Practice, Radiologic Science Education, and Public Interaction
- Radiologic Science Program Standards
- Standards of Education and Regulation for Radiologic Sciences
- State Licensure Examinations by the American Registry of Radiologic Technologists
- Student Membership for Registered Technologists
- Unification of the Profession

American Student Dental Association
<http://www.asdanet.org>

Position/Policy Statements

- Amalgam Restorations
- ASDA Advocacy Program
- Confidentiality of Student Health Status
- Dental School Administrative Policies and Student Government
- Disclosure and Testing of HIV-Positive Status of Health Care Providers
- Due Process
- Ethical Conduct and Professional Behavior of Dental Students
- Faculty-Student Interaction
- Fee for Service
- Fluoridation
- Freedom to Invite Vendors/Speakers
- Hepatitis B Vaccine
- Infection Control Procedures in Audio/Visuals
- Leave of Absence for Dental Students
- National Health Insurance

- Occupational Health and Safety
- Prohibition of Smoking in All Dental School Facilities
- School Closings
- Sensitivity to Diversity
- Sexual Harassment of Dental Students
- Smokeless Tobacco Labeling
- Smoking Ban at ASDA Functions
- Student Involvement in Dental Research
- Student-Sponsored Clinics for the Indigent
- Study Time for National Board Dental Examinations
- Treating Infectious Patients
- Universal Infection Control Procedures
- Use of Animals in Research, Testing, and Education

American Thyroid Association
<http://www.thyroid.org/index.php3>

Position Statement
- Wilson's Syndrome

American Urogynecologic Association
<http://www.augs.org>

Position Statements
- Pelvic Floor Rehabilitation
- Urodynamic Testing

American Urological Association
<http://www.urologyhealth.org/index.cfm>

Policy Statements
- Andrology
- Care of Patients with Urologic Malignancy
- Civil Rights and Professional Responsibility
- Complex Pediatric Urological Care
- Definition of a Urologist
- Definition of Urology
- Delineation of Privileges for ESWL
- Delineation of Privileges for Laparoscopic Urological Procedures
- Delineation of Privileges for Staff Urologists
- Family Medical Leave and Maternity Leave
- Male Sexual Dysfunction
- National Cancer Institute's Physician Data Query
- Osteopathic Physicians

- Patient Requests
- Pediatric Urology
- Productive Work Environment
- Special Interest Areas of Urology
- Urological Allied Health Professionals
- Urologists' Access to New Technology
- Urologists' Use of Imaging Services
- Use of the AUA Logo
- Who Should Practice Urology

Association for Molecular Pathology
<http://www.ampweb.org>

Position Statement
- Recommendations for In-House Development and Operation of Molecular Diagnostic Tests

Association for Professionals in Infection Control and Epidemiology
<http://www.apic.org>

Position Statements
- Hepatitis C Exposure in the Health Care Setting
- Immunization
- Infection Prevention and Control in the Long-Term Care Facility
- Prevention of Device-Mediated Blood-Borne Infections to Health Care Workers
- Release of Nosocomial Infection Data
- Responsibility for Interpretation of the PPD Tuberculin Skin Test
- The Use of Antimicrobial Household Products

Association for Research in Vision and Ophthalmology
<http://www.arvo.org/root/index.asp>

Policy Statements
- Commercial Relationships
- Membership Termination Policy
- Use of Animals in Ophthalmic and Vision Research

Association for the Treatment of Sexual Abusers
<http://www.atsa.com>

Position Statements
- Antiandrogen Therapy and Surgical Castration
- Civil Commitment of Sexually Violent Offenders

- Community Notification Position Statement
- Effective Legal Management of Juvenile Sexual Offenders
- The Importance of Balancing the Need for Research and Participant Protection
- Reducing Sexual Abuse Through Treatment and Intervention with Abusers
- Sexual Abuse As a Public Health Problem

Association of Emergency Physicians
<http://www.aep.org>

Policy and Position Statements

- Access to Emergency Care
- Advance Directives/Living Wills
- Cardiopulmonary Resuscitation
- Certification in Emergency Medicine
- Disaster Emergency Services
- Emergency Care Definition
- Emergency Medicine Definition
- Emergency Physician Definition
- Emergency Physician Qualifications
- Emergency Physician Supply
- EMS Physician Qualifications
- Good Samaritan Status
- Hazardous Materials
- In-Field Medical Director
- Medical Control on Scene
- Medical Direction of Emergency Medical Services
- Off-Line Medical Director
- Online Medical Director
- Prehospital Care by Licensed Practitioners Other Than Physicians
- Prehospital Care Providers Classifications
- Prehospital Defibrillation and AED Use by Non-ALS Personnel
- Prehospital Do-Not-Resuscitate Orders
- Prehospital Thrombolytic Therapy
- Training of Prehospital Care Providers
- Transportation Emergencies in Isolated Surroundings

Association of Maternal and Child Health Programs
<http://amchp.org>

Policy Statements

- Adolescent and School Health

- Children with Special Health Needs
- Data and Assessment
- Service Delivery and Financing
- Teen Pregnancy Prevention
- Women's and Perinatal Health

Association of Nurses in AIDS Care
<http://www.anacnet.org>

Position Statements

- Adolescents and HIV Infection
- Discrimination Protections for People with HIV Infection
- Domestic Partnership Benefits
- Duty to Care
- Endorsement of the AIDS Certified Registered Nurse Credential
- HIV Disease and Tuberculosis
- HIV Reproductive Counseling and Care
- HIV Risk Assessment and Risk Reduction Education
- HIV Serosurveillance and Reporting
- Immigration and HIV Disease
- Maintenance of Disability Benefits for the HIV-Infected Person
- Managed Care
- Medicaid and HIV-Infected Persons
- Medical Use of Marijuana
- Needle and Syringe Exchange
- The Nurse As HIV/AIDS Case Manager
- The Nursing Specialty of HIV/AIDS Care
- Occupational Exposure to HIV Infection and Workers' Compensation
- Palliative Care for Persons Living with HIV/AIDS Including Substance Users
- Postexposure Prophylaxis of Occupational Exposure to HIV Infection
- The Role of Nursing in HIV/AIDS Care
- Substance Use Treatment on Demand

Association of Occupational and Environmental Clinics
<http://aoec.org>

Position Statements

- Asbestos Screening
- Smallpox Vaccination Strategies

Association of Oncology Social Work
<http://www.aosw.org>

Position Papers

- Active Euthanasia and Assisted Suicide
- End-of-Life Care
- Family-Centered Care

Association of Operating Room Nurses
<http://www.aorn.org>

Position Statement

- The Role of Health Care Industry Representatives in the Operating Room

Association of Rehabilitation Nurses
<http://www.rehabnurse.org>

Position Statements

- Advanced Practice in Rehabilitation Nursing
- The Appropriate Inclusion of Rehabilitation Nurses Wherever Rehabilitation Is Provided
- Ethical Issues
- Factors to Consider in Decisions About Staffing in Rehabilitation Nursing Settings
- Inclusion of Rehabilitation Concepts As a Component of Generic Content in BSN Programs
- Rehabilitation of People with Cancer
- The Role of Unlicensed Assistive Personnel in the Rehabilitation Setting

Association of State and Territorial Health Officials
<http://astho.org>

Policy Position Statements

- Access to Health Services
- Comprehensive Environmental Response, Compensation, and Liability Act
- Emerging Infectious Diseases
- Environmental Health Policy Statement
- Health Promotion and Prevention
- HIV/AIDS
- HIV Surveillance
- Immunizations

- Injection Drug Use–Related Blood-Borne Infection
- National Public Health Performance Measurement
- Privacy and Confidentiality of Public Health and Individual Health Data
- Public Health Genetics

Association of Women's Health, Obstetric and Neonatal Nurses
<http://awhonn.org>

Policy Position Statements

- Access to Health Care
- Breast-feeding and Lactation in the Workplace
- Confidentiality in Adolescent Health Care
- Education for Entry into Professional Nursing Practice
- Enhanced Family Medical Leave Protections
- Female Genital Mutilation
- Gender As a Qualification Requirement for Nursing Positions in Women's Health, Obstetric, and Neonatal Nursing
- Health Care Decision Making for Reproductive Care
- HIV Testing and Disclosure for Pregnant Women and Newborns
- Inclusion of Maternal/Newborn Nursing Content in Schools of Nursing
- Infertility Treatment As a Covered Health Insurance Benefit
- Insurance Coverage for Contraceptives
- Interstate Compact for Mutual Recognition of State Licensure
- Midwifery
- National Standards for Newborn Screenings
- Nurses' Rights and Responsibilities Related to Abortion and Sterilization
- Opposition to Mandatory Reporting of Intimate Partner Violence
- Privacy and Confidentiality of Genetic Information
- Protecting the Health of Women and Children from Environmental Toxins
- Rights and Responsibilities of the HIV-Infected Health Care Worker
- The Use of Chaperones During Sensitive Examinations and Treatments
- Women's Health Research

Australasian Society for Ultrasound in Medicine
<http://www.asum.com.au/open/home.htm>

Safety Statements

- Acoustic Output and Equipment Output Display

- Acoustic Streaming
- Continuous-Wave Doppler Fetal Monitoring
- Doppler Ultrasound
- Safety of Ultrasound in Gray-Scale Imaging in Obstetrics
- Thermal Biological Effects
- Ultrasound Contrast Agents

Australasian Society of Clinical Immunology and Allergy
<http://www.allergy.org.au>

Position Papers
- Anaphylaxis in Schools
- Chronic Fatigue Syndrome
- Management of Latex-Allergic Individuals

Australian and New Zealand College of Anaesthetists
<http://www.anzca.edu.au>

Policy Statements
- End-of-Life Decisions
- Infection Control in Anesthesia
- Relief of Pain and Suffering
- Smoking As Related to the Perioperative Period

Australian Institute of Occupational Hygienists
<http://www.aioh.org.au>

Position Paper
- Personal Protective Equipment

Australian Medical Association
<http://www.ama.com.au>

Position Statements
- Access to Medical Records by Doctors Who Are Not Treating the Patients Concerned
- Advertising and Endorsement
- After-Hours Services: Criteria for Deputizing Services
- Alcohol Consumption and Alcohol-Related Problems
- Blood-Borne and Sexually Transmitted Viral Infections
- Boxing
- Breast Cancer Screening
- Breast-feeding

- Care of Older People
- Care of Severely and Terminally Ill Patients
- Certificates Certifying Illness
- Cervical Cancer Screening
- Child Abuse and Neglect
- Code of Ethics
- Definition of Part-Time Work Within the Medical Workforce
- Doctor's Relationships with the Pharmaceutical Industry
- Domestic Violence
- Drugs in Sport
- Endorsement of Products and Services
- Equal Opportunity in the Medical Workforce
- Expert Medical Witnesses: Policy Statements
- Female Genital Mutilation
- Fetal Welfare and the Law
- Firearms
- Guidelines for Doctors Acting As Expert Medical Witnesses
- Guidelines for Doctors on Providing Patient Access to Medical Records
- Health and Medical Research
- Health Care of Prisoners and Detainees
- Health Effects of Problem Gambling

Australian Nursing Council
<http://www.anci.org.au>

Position Statements

- The Inspection of Council Minutes
- Unregulated Workers and Nursing Care

Australian Nursing Federation
<http://www.anf.org.au>

Policies

- Child Care
- Competency Standards and Nursing
- Complementary Therapies in Nursing Practice
- Consultation with ANF in National and/or State/Territory Committees
- Domestic Violence
- Female Genital Mutilation
- Harassment and Victimization in the Workplace

- Information Management and Information Technology
- Management of Nursing and the Nursing Workforce
- Nursing Care
- Nursing Care of the Person Who Is Dying
- Nursing Education
- Occupational Health and Safety
- Organ and Tissue Transplantation
- Peace and Disarmament
- Primary Health Care
- Promoting Breast-feeding
- The Quality Use of Medicine
- Recruitment of Overseas Nurses
- Unpaid Workers in Health Service Agencies

Australian Pain Society
<http://www.apsoc.org.au>

Position Statements
- Epidural Steroids in Chronic Pain
- The Use of Oral Opioids in Patients with Chronic Nonmalignant Pain: Management Strategies

Australian Private Hospitals Association
<http://www.apha.org.au>

Position Statements
- Consumer Choice in Private Health Care
- Contract Negotiations
- Freedom of Choice
- Health Financing

Australian Society of Anesthetists Ltd.
<http://www.asa.org.au>

Policy Documents
- Accreditation
- Infection control
- Informed financial consent

Board of Certification for Emergency Nursing
<http://www.ena.org/bcen>

Position Statements
- Access to Health Care

- Advanced Practice in Emergency Nursing
- Approaching Diversity in Emergency Care
- Autonomous Emergency Nursing Practice
- Blood-Borne Infectious Diseases
- Care of Sexual Assault Victims
- Care of the Critically Ill or Injured Patient During Interfacility Transfer
- Care of the Critically Ill or Injured Patient During Intrafacility Transfer
- Care of the Pediatric Patient During Interfacility Transfer
- Chemical Impairment of Emergency Nurses
- Collaborative and Interdisciplinary Research
- Conscious Sedation
- Customer Service and Satisfaction in the Emergency Department
- Diversity in Emergency Care
- Domestic Violence—Child Maltreatment and Human Neglect
- Educational Recommendations for Nurses Providing Pediatric Emergency Care
- End-of-Life Care in the Emergency Department
- Enhanced 9-1-1 Systems
- Family Presence at the Bedside During Invasive Procedures and/or Resuscitation
- Forensic Evidence Collection
- Hazardous Material Exposure
- Holding Patients in the Emergency Department
- Hospital and Emergency Department Overcrowding
- Injury Prevention
- Integration of Emergency Nursing Concepts in Nursing Curricula
- Latex Allergy
- Mass Casualty Incidents
- Medical Evaluation of Suspected Intoxicated and Psychiatric Patients
- Minimal Trauma Nursing Education Recommendations
- Observation Units
- Obstetrical Patient in the Emergency Department
- Patients with Spontaneous Abortions in the Emergency Department
- Prevention and Treatment of Burns in the Pediatric Population
- Protection of Animal Subjects
- Protection of Human Subjects' Rights
- Resuscitative Decisions
- Role of Delegation by the Emergency Nurse in Clinical Practice Settings

- Role of the Emergency Nurse in Organ and Tissue Donation
- Role of the Registered Nurse in the Prehospital Environment
- Specialty Certification in Emergency Nursing
- Staffing and Productivity in the Emergency Care Setting
- Stress Management Strategies
- Substance Abuse
- Telephone Advice
- Tuberculosis Exposure in the Emergency Department
- The Use of Non-Registered Nurse (Non-RN) Caregivers in Emergency Care
- The Use of the Newly Deceased Patient for Procedural Practice
- Violence in the Emergency Care Setting
- Voluntary Smallpox Vaccination
- Weapons of Mass Destruction

Brain Injury Association of America
<http://www.biausa.org/Pages/home.html>

Issue Briefs
- Education Reform
- Family Opportunity Act
- Mental Health Parity
- MiCASSA
- Patient's Bill of Rights

British Association of Paediatric Surgeons
<http://www.baps.org.uk>

Policy Documents of the Ethics Committee
- Androgen Insensitivity Syndrome
- Cloning
- Considerations Relating to How Much to Tell Parents, Patients/Children
- Male Ritual Circumcision
- Ownership of Excised Tissue and Implants
- Withdrawing and Withholding Treatment

British Columbia College of Family Physicians
<http://www.bccfp.bc.ca>

Position Paper
- Primary Care and Family Medicine

British Columbia Medical Association
<http://www.bcma.org/Index.htm>

Policy Papers and Reports

- Attracting and Retaining Physicians in Rural British Columbia
- Capitation: A Wolf in Sheep's Clothing?
- Evaluation of Rostering Patients
- Managed Care
- Obtaining Effective Medical Input into Regional Decision Making
- Regionalization of Health Care
- Saving Medicare for Canadians
- Wait List Report II

Issues and Backgrounders

- CMA Survey on Specialty Care Capacity
- Comparison of Compensation Increases in Health Care in BC
- Electronic Medical Records
- Establishing Medically Required and Core Services
- Federal Transfer Payments
- Health Care Access
- Health Care Funding
- How Physicians in BC Are Compensated
- Medicare's Future
- Pharmacare Financing Options
- Physician Supply
- Primary Care Demonstration Projects
- Primary Care Reform
- Protecting the Privacy of Personal Health Information
- Regional Health Care Funding Formula

British Columbia Society of Occupational Therapists
<http://www.bcsot.org>

Position Statements

- BCSOT Role in a Changing Health Care System
- Educating Occupational Therapists in BC

British Dietetic Association
<http://www.bda.uk.com>

Position Papers and Statements

- Continuing Professional Development for Dietitians
- Dietary Treatment of People with High Coronary Risk

- High-Protein, Low-Carbohydrate Diets
- Hospital Food As Treatment
- Malnutrition in Hospitals
- Medical and Clinical Audit
- Obesity
- Peanut Allergy
- Phytoestrogens in Soya Infant Formula
- Setting and Monitoring Standards in the Workplace
- Vitamins and Minerals

British Fertility Society
<http://www.britishfertilitysociety.org.uk>

Policy Statements
- In Vitro Maturation of Oocytes
- Preimplantation Diagnosis

British Geriatrics Society
<http://www.bgs.org.uk>

Guidelines, Policy Statements, and Statements of Good Practice
- Model Workload for Consultants in Geriatric Medicine
- NHS Medical Services for Older People—Advice to Commissioners and Providers
- Rehabilitation of Older People
- Standards of Medical Care for Older People—Expectations and Recommendations

Health Promotion
- Acute Medical Care for Elderly People
- Collaboration Between Physicians of Geriatric Medicine and Psychiatrists of Old Age
- Collaboration with Other Specialties
- Continence Care—A Guide for those Working in Residential and Nursing Homes
- The Discharge of Elderly Persons from Hospital for Community Care
- Domiciliary Assessment Visits
- The Elderly Patient in the A&E Department
- Geriatric Day Hospitals and Ambulatory Care
- Interface Between Hospital and Community
- Intermediate Care—Medical Guidance for Purchasers and Providers

- Policy for Health Promotion and Preventive Care for Older People
- Seamless Care—Obstacles and Solutions

Community, Private, and Independent Sector

- The Assessment of Frail Elderly People Being Considered for or in Receipt of Continuing Care
- Work of the Geriatrician in the Community

Training and Manpower

- BGS Training Committee Recommended Reading List
- Core Content of Postgraduate Curriculum in Elderly Care Medicine
- Core Content of Undergraduate Curriculum in Elderly Care Medicine
- General Practitioner Vocational Training in Geriatric Medicine
- Syllabus in Psychiatry in Old Age for Trainees in Geriatric Medicine
- Training in Geriatric Medicine

Ethics and Law

- The Abuse of Older People
- Advice on Cardiopulmonary Resuscitation Policies
- British Geriatrics Society Guidelines on Testamentary Capacity
- Guidelines on Artificial Hydration and Nutrition in Elderly Patients
- Procedures for Compulsory Admissions of Patients Without Acute Purely Psychiatric Illness

British Medical Association

<http://www.bma.org.uk/ap.nsf/Content/splashpage>

Policies

- Abortion
- Access to Health Care
- Adolescent Health Issues
- Advertising
- Age of Consent
- Aircraft
- Alcohol
- All Work Tests
- Alternative Therapies
- Ancillary Staff and Remedial Professions
- Annual Report of Council
- Armed Forces
- Arms

- Artificial Limb and Appliance Centre
- Awards and Honours
- Biotechnology
- Blood Transfusion Service
- BMA Charities
- BMA Policy
- BMJ Publishing Group
- Boxing
- British Medical Journal
- Business of the ARM
- Bylaws
- Cancer Screening
- Careers
- Care of the Dying
- Car Parking
- Certification
- Charities
- Charles Hastings Wine Club
- Child Abuse
- Child Care Facilities
- Child Health Care
- Clinical Audit
- Clinical Governance
- Clinical Indicators
- Clinical Responsibility
- Community Care
- Competitive Tendering
- Complaints Procedures
- Confidentiality
- Consent to Treatment
- Constitution of the Association
- Council
- Deputising Services
- Devolution
- Disabled Persons
- Disciplinary Procedures
- Doctors' Performance
- Dogs
- Driving Licensing
- Drug, Alcohol, and Solvent Abuse
- Drugs
- Emergency Services

- Environment
- Ethical Research Committees
- European Community
- Euthanasia
- Extracontractual Referrals
- Family Planning
- Fellows
- Female Circumcision
- Finances of the Association
- First Aid
- Food
- Forensic Medicine
- Freedom of Speech
- Function, Structure, and Funding of the NHS
- Funding
- General Medical Council
- General Practice
- Genetic Engineering
- Geriatrics
- Health Education
- Health Strategy
- Hepatitis B
- HIV/AIDS
- Hospital Services
- Human Rights and Discrimination
- Information Technology
- Insurance Companies
- International Affairs
- International Medical Associations
- Intimate Body Searches
- Intraprofessional Conflicts
- Junior Hospital Staff
- League Tables
- Library
- London
- Management
- Maternity Care
- Medical Academic Staff
- Medical Advisory Machinery
- Medical Education
- Medical Ethics
- Medical Negligence

- Medical Students
- Medical Workforce
- Medicine and the Law
- Mental Health
- Mileage Allowances
- Millennium
- Morale
- National Health Service
- National Institute for Clinical Excellence and Commission for Health Improvement
- No-Fault Compensation
- Northern Ireland
- Nuclear Power/War
- Nursing
- Obstetrics
- Occupational Health
- Ophthalmic Medical Services
- Overseas Doctors
- Parental Benefits
- Part-Time Work
- Patient's Charter
- Performance Indicators
- Prescribing
- President
- Primary Care Groups
- Priority Setting
- Prison
- Private Finance Initiative
- Private Medical Care
- Private Practice and Professional Fees
- Professional Affinity Group Services Limited
- Professional Indemnity
- The Public Health
- Public Health Medicine and Community Health
- Purchaser/Provider Arrangements
- Purchasing and Commissioning
- Quality of Care
- Rabies
- Rape and Sexual Abuse
- Rationing
- Rehabilitation and Resuscitation
- Remuneration and DDRB

- Report by Chairman of Council
- Report of the Agenda Committee
- Representative Body
- Research
- Road Safety
- Safety in Clinical Practice
- Scientific Activities
- Scotland
- Seasonal Pressures
- Secondary to Primary Care Shift
- Secretariat
- Senior Hospital Doctors
- Services to Members
- Sex Selection
- Sick Doctors
- Smoking
- Social Services
- Sport
- Structure and Function of the BMA
- Study Leave
- Superannuation
- Terms and Conditions of Service
- Toxic Substances
- Trades Union Congress
- Training and Education
- Transplant of Human Organs
- Transport and Health
- Transport of Patients
- Violence
- Wales
- Welsh Language Act
- Women Doctors

British Society for Human Genetics
<http://www.bshg.org.uk>

Official Statements

- Arrangements for Genetic Testing for Rare Disorders
- Commissioning Specialised Services
- Genetic Testing and Insurance
- Genetic Testing of Children
- Joint Statement on Genetic Research and Insurance

- Patenting and Clinical Genetics
- Patenting Human Gene Sequences
- Prenatal Detection of Aneuploidy
- The Role of the Clinical Geneticist

British Toxicology Society
<http://www.thebts.org>

Position Statements
- EU White Paper: Strategy for a Future Chemicals Policy
- Herbal Medicines

British Transplantation Society
<http://www.bts.org.uk>

Position Statement
- Paired Organ Exchange

California Academy of Family Physicians
<http://www.familydocs.org>

Issues Monographs
- Family Physicians and Inpatient Care in the Era of the Hospitalist
- Family Physicians: The Logical Resource for Our Changing Health Care Environment
- Making the Most of Physician-Patient E-mail
- Welcome to Your First Year in Practice

California Society of Pathologists
<http://www.calpath.org>

Position Statements
- PAP Smear Review Policy Statement
- Pathologist Professional Component Billing for Clinical Pathology Services

Canadian Academy of Sport Medicine
<http://www.casm-acms.org>

Position Statements
- Bicycle Helmet Safety
- Body Composition
- Concussions
- Exercise in Pregnancy

- Facial Protection in Hockey
- Gender Verification
- HIV in Sport
- Violence in Hockey

Canadian Anesthesiologists' Society
<http://www.cas.ca>

Position Statements
- Preadmission Clinics in Anesthesia

Canadian Association of Critical Care Nurses
<http://www.caccn.ca>

Position Statements
- Nonregulated Health Personnel in Critical Care Areas
- Withholding and Withdrawing of Life Support

Canadian Association of Emergency Physicians
<http://www.caep.ca>

Position Statements
- Emergency Department Overcrowding
- Informed Consent for Emergency Procedures
- Public Access Defibrillation Programs
- Steroids in Acute Spinal Cord Injury
- Taking of Blood Alcohol Levels in the Emergency Department
- Ultrasonography in the Emergency Department
- Writing of Patient Admission Orders

Canadian Association of General Surgeons
<http://www.cags-accg.ca>

Position Statements
- Ambulatory Care
- On-Call time for General Surgeons

Canadian Association of Interns and Residents
<http://www.cair.ca>

Position Papers
- Communicable Diseases
- Discussion Paper—Return of Service
- International Medical Graduates

- The New Face of Medicine: Sustaining and Enhancing Medicine
- Physician Resources 1 and 2
- Recruitment and Retention of Physicians
- Recruitment and Retention of Physicians to Nonurban Practice Areas
- Resident Intimidation and Harassment
- Resident Well-Being
- The Response of the Canadian Association of Interns and Residents to the Report

Canadian Association of Occupational Therapists
<http://www.caot.ca>

Position Statements

- The Agreement on Internal Trade
- Continuing Professional Education
- Everyday Occupations and Health
- Health Promotion
- International Marketing
- Joint Position Statement on Evidence-Based Occupational Therapy
- Occupational Therapy and Ergonomics
- Support Personnel in Occupational Therapy Services

Canadian Association of Paediatric Surgeons
<http://www.caps.ca>

Position Statement

- Pediatric Constipation—Guidelines for Referral to a Pediatric Surgeon

Canadian Association of Physicians for the Environment
<http://www.cape.ca>

Position Statements

- Acid Deposition and Transregional Pollution
- Ambient Air Quality
- Biodiversity
- Breast Cancer
- Genetically Modified Organisms Statement from CAPE
- The Greenhouse Effect and Global Climate Change
- Indoor Air Quality
- Lead Exposure and Health Effects

- Population Growth and Sustainable Development
- Stratospheric Ozone Depletion and Enhanced Exposure to Ultraviolet Irradiation
- Sustainable Development
- Why Canadian Physicians Are Concerned About the Policies Regulating Pesticide Use

Canadian Association of Radiation Oncologists
<http://www.caro-acro.ca>

Position Statements
- Access to Treatment
- Physician/Industry Relationship Guidelines
- Specialist Certification in Radiation Oncology

Canadian Cardiovascular Society
<http://www.ccs.ca>

Position Statements/Public Policy
- Current Issues in Cardiac Transplantation: Strategies to Improve Organ Donation
- Grading of Angina/Classification de l'Angine de Poitrine
- Use of Sildenafil in the Management of Sexual Dysfunction

Canadian Chiropractic Association
<http://www.ccachiro.org>

Position Statements
- Chiropractic Care for Infants, Children, and Adolescents
- Orthopractic and Other Nonregulated Groups
- Vaccination and Immunization

Canadian College of Medical Geneticists
<http://ccmg.medical.org>

Policy Statements
- Banking Guidelines
- Cystic Fibrosis Testing/Screening
- Genetic Testing of Minors
- Prenatal Diagnosis Guidelines
- Prenatal Paternity Testing

Canadian Healthcare Association
<http://www.cha.ca>

Position Paper

- Preventing and Resolving Ethical Conflicts Involving Health Care Providers and Persons Receiving Care

Canadian Infectious Disease Society
<http://www.cids.medical.org>

Position Statements

- Anthrax
- *E. coli* O157/H7-Related Diseases
- HIV Screening of Individuals Applying for Canadian Immigrant Status, and Acceptance/Exclusion of Persons Found to Be HIV-Positive
- Hospital-Acquired Infections
- Human Immunodeficiency Virus and Drug Resistance Influenza
- Legionella Pneumonia
- Malaria and Other Imported Diseases in Canadian Travelers
- Meningococcal Infections and Meningitis
- Methicillin-Resistant Staphylococcus aureus
- Needle Sticks in the Community
- Pneumococcal Vaccine to Prevent Pneumonia Cryptosporidiosis
- Spreading of Sewage Sludge on Agricultural Lands

Canadian Medical Association
<http://www.cma.ca>

Policy Statements

- Approaches to Enhancing the Quality of Drug Therapy
- CMA Charter for Physicians
- CMA Health Information Privacy Code
- Core and Comprehensive Health Care Services
- Determining Medical Fitness to Drive
- Environmentally Responsible Activity in the Health Sector
- Euthanasia and Assisted Suicide
- Federal Health Financing
- Fetal Alcohol Syndrome
- Firearms Control
- The Future of Medicine
- Guidelines for Assessing Health System Performance
- HIV Infection in the Workplace

- Joint Statement on Preventing and Resolving Ethical Conflicts
- Joint Statement on Resuscitation Interventions
- The Medical Record: Confidentiality, Access, and Disclosure
- Medication Use and the Elderly
- Natural Health Products
- Obstetric Care
- Operational Principles for the Measurement and Management of Waiting Lists
- Organ and Tissue Donation and Transplantation
- The Patient-Physician Relationship and the Sexual Abuse of Patients
- The Physician Appointment and Reappointment Process
- Physician Compensation
- Physician Health and Well-Being
- Physician Resource Planning
- Physicians and the Pharmaceutical Industry
- Prevention of Transmission of Hepatitis B
- Principles for Medical Care of Older Persons
- Principles for Reentry System in Canadian Postgraduate Medical Education
- Regionalization
- The Role of Physicians in Prevention and Health Promotion
- Rural and Remote Practice Issues
- Statement of Principles: The Sale and Use of Data on Individual Physician's Prescribing
- Tobacco and Health

Canadian Nurses Association
<http://www.cna-nurses.ca/cna>

Position Statements

Education
- Doctoral and Postdoctoral Preparation in Nursing
- Education of Health and Social Service Professionals in Gerontology and Geriatrics
- Education Support for Competent Nursing Practice
- Ethical Nursing Recruitment
- Human Rights
- Prevention and Resolving Ethical Conflicts Involving Health Care Providers
- Privacy of Personal Health Information

- Resuscitative Interventions
- Screening for Alcohol or Drugs in the Workplace

Health and Finance
- Financing Canada's Health System
- Framework for Canada's Health System
- Pay Equity

Health Public Policy
- Environmentally Responsible Activity

Leadership
- Clinical Nurse Specialist
- Interdisciplinary Approach in Continuing Care
- The Nurse Practitioner
- Nursing Leadership

Primary Health Care
- Food Safety and Security Are Determinants of Health
- International Trade and Labour Mobility
- Joint CFPC/CNA Position Statement on Physical Activity
- Mental Health Care Reform
- Nursing Professional Regulatory Framework
- Peace and Security
- Reducing the Use of Tobacco Products
- Substance Misuse and Chemical Dependency by Nurses
- Tobacco: The Role of Health Professionals in Smoking Cessation Protection of the Public
- Unregulated Health Care Workers Supporting Nursing Care Delivery

Research
- Collecting Data to Reflect the Impact of Nursing Practice
- Evidence-Based Decision Making and Nursing Practice

Canadian Ophthalmological Society
<http://www.eyesite.ca>

Policies and Position Statement
- Appropriate Referral
- Commercial Tanning Facilities
- Contact Lenses
- Delegation to Paramedical Personnel
- Eye Banks
- Eye Care

- Glaucoma and the Use of Marijuana
- Health Care and Governments
- HIV/AIDS and the Eye
- Independent Departments of Ophthalmology
- Learning Disabilities, Dyslexia, and Vision
- Low Vision
- Optometric Use of Drugs for Therapeutic Purposes
- Postoperative Eye Care
- Prophylactic Management of Gonococcal Ophthalmia
- Relationship of Ophthalmology and Optometry
- Role of Ophthalmology
- Spectacle-Mounted Telescopes for Driving
- Ultrasonography of the Eye and Orbit
- Ultraviolet Radiation and the Eye
- Use of Ophthalmic Drugs by Nonphysicians
- Video Display Terminal Risk

Canadian Paediatric Society
<http://www.cps.ca>

Position Papers

- Adolescent Medicine
- Adolescent Pregnancy
- Age Limits and Adolescence
- Care of the Chronically Ill Adolescent
- Eating Disorders in Adolescents: Principles of Diagnosis and Treatment
- Emergency Contraception
- Family-Friendly Adolescent Health Care
- Health Care Standards for Youth in Custodial Facilities
- Office Practice Guidelines for the Care of Adolescents
- Prevention of Firearm Deaths in Canadian Children and Adolescents
- Sexual Abuse of Adolescents with Chronic Conditions

Canadian Pain Society
<http://www.canadianpainsociety.com>

Position Statements

- Pain Relief
- Use of Opioid Analgesics for the Treatment of Chronic Noncancer Pain

Canadian Pharmacists Association
<http://www.pharmacists.ca/index.cfm>

Position Statements

- Breast-feeding and Infant Nutrition
- CMA/CPhA Joint Statement—Approaches to Enhancing the Quality of Drug Therapy
- CPhA Position Statement on Direct-to-Consumer Advertising
- Direct-to-Consumer Advertising
- Ethics of Relationships Between Pharmacists and Pharmaceutical Manufacturers
- The Pharmacist with HIV/AIDS
- Public Confusion Resulting from Line Extensions
- Role of the Pharmacist in Preventing and Limiting the Transmission of HIV and the Spread of AIDS
- Tobacco

Canadian Psychiatric Association
<http://www.cpa-apc.org>

Position Statements

- Access to New Medications
- Adult Recovered Memories of Childhood Sexual Abuse
- Biofeedback
- Clozapine
- The Confidentiality of Psychiatric Records and the Patient's Right to Privacy
- Corporal Punishment of Children
- Current Status of Megavitamin and Orthomolecular Therapies
- Definition of Psychotherapy
- Environmental Hypersensitivity
- Guidelines on Ethics in Courtroom Testimony
- HIV Disease
- Hunger Strikes in the Correctional Service of Canada
- Prozac
- Psychiatric Bed Levels
- Sexual Misconduct

Position Papers and Guidelines

- Assaultive and Destructive Behaviour in a Treatment Setting
- The CMA Code of Ethics Annotated for Psychiatrists
- Curriculum Guidelines for Residency Training Psychiatrists in Substance-Related Disorders

- Evidence-Based Psychiatric Practice
- Guidelines Covering Professional Conduct for Psychiatrists in Penitentiary Services
- Guidelines for Phase IV Clinical Trials
- Human Resources in Psychiatry
- Placebos in Clinical Trials of Psychotropic Medications
- Psychosurgery
- The Role of Psychiatrists in Quality Review
- Shared Mental Health Care in Canada
- Teaching on Gender Issues
- Treatment of the Mentally Ill Physician
- Unilateral Termination of Treatment by a Psychiatrist

Canadian Public Health Association
<http://www.cpha.ca>

Policy Statements

- A Brief Regarding Bill C-68 As It Relates to Public Health
- The Canada Health and Social Transfer and Health Equity in Canada
- Creating Conditions for Health
- Federal/Provincial/Territorial Arrangements for Health Policy
- Focus on Health: Public Health in Health Services Restructuring
- The Future of Public Health in Canada
- Health Impacts of Social and Economic Conditions: Implications for Public Policy
- HIV/AIDS: A Public Health Perspective
- Human and Ecosystem Health: Canadian Perspectives, Canadian Actions
- Joint Statement on Shaken Baby Syndrome
- National Leadership for Public Health Research in the 1990s
- An Ounce of Prevention: Strengthening the Balance in Health Care Reform
- Public Health and the Blood System in Canada
- Statement on Peace, Security, and Public Health
- Violence in Society: A Public Health Perspective

Other Papers

- Action Statement for Health Promotion in Canada
- Discussion Paper on the Health Impact of Unemployment
- Environment and Health: Linked for Life
- Position Paper on Homelessness and Health

- Public Health Infrastructure in Canada
- SPHA Series of Articles on Health Determinants
- Sustainability and Equity: Primary Health Care in Developing Countries

Canadian Society for International Health
<http://www.csih.org>

Position Papers

- Economic Globalization, Trade Liberalization, Governance, and Health
- A Global Tobacco Treaty
- Peace and Health

Canadian Society for Pharmaceutical Sciences
<http://cspscanada.org>

Consultation/Position Papers

- Changes to the Authority to Sell Drugs
- Fees Regulations
- Prohibited Substances: Proposal to Amend the Food and Drug Regulations
- Standards for Comparative Claims Related to Therapeutic Aspects of Drugs

Canadian Society of Addiction Medicine
<http://www.csam.org>

Policy Statements

- Definitions in Addiction Medicine
- Harm Reduction
- Medicinal Use of Cannabis
- Statement on National Drug Policy
- Use of Opioids for Chronic Nonmalignant Pain

Canadian Society of Allergy and Clinical Immunology
<http://csaci.medical.org>

Position Statements

- Allergy Skin Testing
- Clinical Ecology
- Dangers of Sulfating Agents in Food and Pharmaceuticals
- Food Labeling by Restaurants and Caterers

- Intraocular Pressure and Inhaled Corticosteroids
- Nonprescription Availability of Theophylline, Epinephrine, and Ephedrine for Asthma
- Risks of Asthma and Anaphylaxis During ß-Blocker Therapy
- Smoking in the Home by Parents of Asthmatic Children

Canadian Society of Hospital Pharmacists
<http://www.cshp.ca>

Position Statements
- Institutional Pharmacy Research
- Monitoring Drug Therapy in the Elderly
- Pharmaceutical Care
- The Pharmacist's Role in Home Health Care
- Size, Shape, and Color of Medications

Canadian Society of Nuclear Medicine
<http://www.csnm.medical.org>

Policy Statement
- Standards for Positron Emission Tomography

Position Statement
- Medical Use of Positron-Emitting Agents in Canada

Canadian Urological Association
<http://www.cua.org>

Position Statements
- Asymptomatic Microscopic Hematuria
- Investigation and Management of Antenatal-Detected Hydronephrosis
- Minimal-Access Surgery
- Prostate-Specific Antigen
- The Workup of Azoospermic Males

Catholic Health Association of Canada
<http://www.chac.ca>

Position Papers
- Advance Health Care Directives
- Social Policy

Position Briefs

- Euthanasia and Assisted Suicide
- Organ Donation
- Palliative Care
- Reproductive Technology

College of American Pathologists
<http://www.cap.org/apps/cap.portal>

Public Policy

- Accreditation
- Acquired Immunodeficiency Syndrome
- Autopsy
- Blood and Blood Banking
- Clinical Laboratory Improvement Amendments
- Cytopathology
- Fraud and Abuse
- Genetic Medicine
- Guidelines
- Health Care Delivery
- Health Education
- Health Insurance
- Health System Reform
- Health Workforce
- Pap Test
- Pathologic Specimens
- Patient Safety
- Payment and Reimbursement
- Scope of Practice
- Self-Referral
- Standards
- Tissue and Organ Donation

College of Family Physicians of Canada
<http://www.cfpc.ca/global/splash/default.asp?s=1>

Policies, Reports, and Position Statements

- Our Strength for Tomorrow: Valuing Our Children
- Primary Care and Family Medicine in Canada: A Prescription for Renewal

Endorsed by the College of Family Physicians of Canada

- Canada's Guide to Healthy Physical Activity
- Guidelines for Childhood Immunization Practices

- Guidelines on Red Blood Cell and Plasma Transfusion in Adults and Children
- Routine Administration of Vitamin K to Newborns
- Violence Against Women Empower Education Program

College of Physicians and Surgeons of Alberta
<http://www.cpsa.ab.ca/home/home.asp>

Policies and Guidelines

- Advertising by Physicians
- After-Hours Availability of Physicians
- Alberta Physicians' Involvement in Planned Domiciliary Deliveries
- Basic Obstetrics in Alberta Hospitals
- Charging for Uninsured Services
- Cleaning, Disinfecting, and Sterilizing Office Instruments
- Collection of Blood in Physicians' Offices
- Colposcopy and Laser Surgery of the Lower Genital Tract
- Competency Assessment and Surrogate Decision Making
- Conflict of Interest
- Doctor/Patient Sexual Involvement
- Elective Cardioversion for Atrial Fibrillation
- Facsimile Transmission of Prescriptions
- Gynecologic Operative Endoscopy
- Hepatitis B Virus Infection in Health Care Workers
- HIV Infection in Health Care Workers
- Laser Surgery
- Management of Chronic Nonmalignant Pain
- Medical Examinations by Nontreating Physicians
- Opting Out of the Publicly Funded Health Care System
- Physician/Patient Relationships
- Physicians' Office Medical Records
- Practice in Association
- Preventing Follow-up Failures When Caring for Patients
- Principles of Ownership
- Reentry into Practice
- The Referral/Consultation Process
- Release of Medical Information
- Reporting to the College
- Reporting Unfit Drivers
- Resuscitation and Care of Critically Ill Newborns
- Termination of Pregnancy
- Visiting Surgery/Anesthesia

College of Physicians and Surgeons of British Columbia
<http://www.cpsbc.ca/cps>

Position Statements

- BC Palliative Care Benefits, Program Description, and Application
- Benzodiazepines and Other Targeted Substances Regulations
- Evidence-Based Recommendations for Medical Management of Chronic Nonmalignant Health Care Consent Legislation
- Manual for the Accreditation of Nonhospital Medical/Surgical Facilities
- Medical Practitioners Act
- Medical Professionalism in the New Millennium: A Physician Charter
- Pain Guidance Document for Practitioners
- Payment for Sexual Assault Medical Forensic Evidence
- The Prevention of Cross Infection in the Physician's Office
- Rules Made Under the Medical Practitioners Act
- Standards for Nonhospital Medical Hyperbaric Oxygen Facilities
- Task Force on Physician Supply in Canada
- Use of Selective Serotonin Reuptake Inhibitors in Children

College of Physicians and Surgeons of Manitoba
<http://www.cpsm.mb.ca>

Guidelines and Statements

- Anaesthesia
- Diagnostic Imaging
- Ethics and Administration
- Laboratory Medicine
- Licensure/Qualifications
- Medicine
- Nuclear Medicine
- Ophthalmology
- Paediatrics
- Pharmacy
- Psychiatry
- Surgery
- Women's Health

College of Physicians and Surgeons of New Brunswick
<http://www.cpsnb.org>

Guidelines

- Breast Examination
- Charging for Uninsured Services
- Confidentiality and Release of Information
- Guidelines for Management of Chronic Nonmalignant Pain
- The Patient Medical Record
- Patient Privacy—Examinations Respecting Privacy
- Reporting of Colleagues
- Sexuality in the Physician/Patient Relationship

College of Physicians and Surgeons of Nova Scotia
<http://www.cpsns.ns.ca>

Guidelines and Policies

- Conflict of Interest Guidelines
- Controlled Substances: Ethical Issues
- Controlled Substances: Legal Issues
- General Guidelines for Office Procedures Where Conscious Sedation Is Required
- Guidelines for Medical-Legal Reports
- Guidelines for the Provision of Telemedicine Services
- Guidelines for the Use of Controlled Substances in the Treatment of Pain
- Policy on Physician Withdrawal of Services During Job Actions
- Selling Products Out of the Office
- Sexual Misconduct in the Physician-Patient Relationship

College of Physicians and Surgeons of Ontario
<http://www.cpso.on.ca>

Policy Statements

- Avoid Complaints of Sexual Abuse
- Block Fees
- Complementary Medicine
- Confidentiality and Access to Patient Information
- Conflict of Interest
- Consent to Medical Treatment
- Cooperation with the College
- Delegation of Controlled Acts
- Drugs and Prescribing Group of Policies

- Ending the Physician-Patient Relationship
- Female Circumcision, Excision, and Infibulation
- Guarantor for Change of Name
- Guidelines for Supervision of Medical Students
- Mandatory Reporting
- MDs' Relations with Drug Companies
- Medical Records
- Physician-Patient "Dating"
- Prescribing Medical Marijuana
- Professional Misconduct
- Requirements When Changing Scope of Practice
- Requirements When Reentering Medical Practice
- Supervision of Postgraduate Trainees
- Syringe Disposal
- Third-Party Medical Reports
- Treatment of Patients by Medical Students and Postgraduate Trainees
- Vaccine Storage
- Withdrawal of Physician Services During Job Action

College of Physicians and Surgeons of Saskatchewan
<http://www.quadrant.net/cpss>

Policies and Guidelines

- Acupuncture
- AIDS/HIV Infection Policy
- Anaesthesia/Analgesia—Obstetrical
- Anaesthesia—Guidelines to Practice
- Anaesthesia—Postanaesthesia Recovery Room
- Anaesthesia—Privileges (Less than 100 beds)
- Anaesthesia—Training Requirements
- Audit—Guidelines for Medical Audit
- Blood Transfusion Services—Use of Local Donors
- Bylaw—Procedures Conducted in Nonhosp. Medical/Surgical Facilities
- Bylaws—College of Physicians and Surgeons
- Bylaws—Health Care Facilities Credentialing Committee
- Cancer—Sask. Cancer Foundation Policies
- Colposcopy
- Credentialing Guidelines—Hospitals Less than 100 beds
- C-Section—Preventing/Ensuring Indications
- Day Surgery

- Day Surgery and Anaesthesia Guidelines
- Death—Policy on Pronouncement
- Desamethasone, detamethasone—*see* Tocolytic Drugs
- Drug Research—Criteria to Guide Physician Participation in Clinical Drug Research
- ECG Guidelines
- Epidural Anaesthesia/Analgesic Guidelines
- Exercise ECG Testing
- Gestational Diabetes
- Glasgow Coma Scale
- Head Injury Protocol—Lloydminster Hospital
- Hepatitis B Policy
- Hospital Standards Act
- House Call Service from Saskatoon
- Induction—Syntocinon—Protocol
- Infection Control and Waste Management in Physicians' Offices
- Insemination—Therapeutic Donor Guidelines
- Intracervical Prostaglandin Gel
- Intravaginal Prostaglandin Gel
- Investigation of Members—College Policy in Response to Public Inquiries
- Laparoscopic Cholecystectomy
- Laparoscopic Tubal Ligation
- Malignant Hyperthermia
- Mammography Interpretation Eligibility
- Management of Chronic Nonmalignant Pain
- Medi-Clinics
- Midwifery—Nonmedical
- Neonatal Resuscitation Guidelines—National
- Newsletter—Editorial Policy
- Nonionic Contrast Media
- Nonionic Contrast Media—Draft Guideline
- Nonresident Physicians—Privileges
- Nuclear Medicine Credentialing
- Obstetrics—Assessing Skills and Knowledge
- Obstetrics—Guidelines for Performance of Ultrasound
- Obstetrics—Number of Deliveries to Maintain
- Operative Endoscopy—Specialty of O/G
- Opioids—Criteria for Prescribing
- Orthopaedics—Assessing Skills and Knowledge
- Peer Support and Review Program
- Physician at Risk to Patients—Policy

- Physicians at Risk
- Postgraduate Clinical Trainees—Supervision
- (Prostin E2) Protocol—Replace Syntocinon
- Provision of CPPS Services to Outside Agencies
- Radiological Supervision at Medi-Centres
- Radiology—Standards of Practice
- Retraining for Eligibility
- Sick Leave for Pregnancy
- Sick Slips
- Small Hospital Follow-up Management
- Stillbirth—Autopsy
- Stillbirth—Guidelines for Management of Patients
- Streptococcal Infections in the Newborn
- Streptokinase—*see* Thrombolytic Therapy Protocol
- Surgery—Responsibility in Postoperative Care
- Thrombolytic Therapy Protocol
- Tocolytic Drugs for Maternal Transport
- Tonsillectomy Guidelines
- Training to Perform Ultrasound
- Transfusion Practice Guidelines
- Ultrasound—Antepartum Obstetrical Exam Guidelines
- Ultrasound—Qualifications for Payment
- Ultrasound—Reporting of Obstetrical
- Ultrasound—Review
- Unproven and Unconventional Treatment
- Usage of High Osmolar Contrast Media
- Walk-in Clinics—Ethical Operation

College on Problems of Drug Dependence
<http://www.cpdd.vcu.edu>

Position Statements

- National Drug Policy
- Research with Laboratory Animals
- Tobacco

Research Advances Fact Sheets

- Behavioral and Psychosocial Treatments for Drug Abuse
- Drug Abuse Research and the Health of the Nation
- Medication Treatments for Drug Abuse

Colorado Health and Hospital Association
<http://www.cha.com>

Position Statements

- Breathing Matters
- Cesarean Delivery
- Childhood Immunization in Colorado
- Containing Health Care Costs
- The Cost of Violence
- Injuries Are No Accident
- The Silent Epidemic: Women and Heart Disease
- Teenage Pregnancy
- Tobacco and Health
- Update on Violence and Teenage Pregnancy

Colorado Medical Society
<http://www.cms.org>

Position and Concept Papers

- Individually Owned, Individually Selected Health Care
- Medicaid
- Medicare Transformation
- Physician Affiliation/Disaffiliation
- Physicians' Specific Data
- Transition of Care

Congress of Neurological Surgeons
<http://www.neurosurgeon.org>

Position Statements

- Bone Dowels from Human Tissue
- Placebo Surgery
- Placement of Intracranial Pressure Monitors by Midlevel Practitioners in Neurotrauma and Emergency Neurosurgical Care

Council of State and Territorial Epidemiologists
<http://www.cste.org>

Position Statements

- Access to and Dissemination of NPHSS Data
- Adding Acute Pesticide Poisoning/Injuries (APP/I) As a Condition Reportable to the National Public Health Surveillance System
- Adding Ehrlichiosis As a Condition Reportable to the NPHSS

- Adding Elevated Blood Lead Levels Among Adults As a Condition Reportable to the National Public Health Surveillance System
- Adding Elevated Blood Lead Levels Among Young Children As a Condition Reportable to the National Public Health Surveillance System
- Adding Giardiasis As a Nationally Notifiable Disease
- Adding Silicosis As a Condition Reportable to the National Public Health Surveillance System (NPHSS)
- Addition of Listeriosis to the List of Nationally Notifiable Diseases
- Addressing Lymphatic Filariasis in States and U.S. Territories
- Airline TB Contact Notifications
- Assessing the Importance of Motorcycle Helmet Laws
- Asthma Surveillance and Case Definition
- Asthma Surveillance Projects
- Availability of Affordable Human Rabies Vaccine
- Bicycle Helmets
- Birth Defect Surveillance
- Bone Infections Associated with Injection Drug Use
- Cataloging current state chronic disease programs
- CDC-Developed Surveillance Software
- CDC Initiative for the Prevention and Control of Disease, Injury, and Disability in Child Care Settings
- CDC Initiative on Emerging Infectious Diseases
- CDC to Seek New Funding for Communicable Disease Control Programs in Inner Cities and Other High Disease Incidence Areas
- Changes in the Case Definition for Human Ehrlichiosis, and Addition of a New Ehrlichiosis Category As a Condition Placed Under Surveillance According to the National Public Health Surveillance System (NPHSS)
- Cholera
- Chronic Disease Program Integration
- Chronic Hepatitis B Virus Infection
- Close CSTE Affiliations with ASTPHLD
- Collection of Health and Risk Factor Data in Schools
- Communicating the Unique Role of Public Health in Injury Prevention
- Comprehensive Asthma Surveillance and Prevention Program
- Comprehensive Surveillance Plan
- Consideration of Pesticide Residues in Water Quality Assessment
- Continuation of Cryptosporidiosis Under National Surveillance
- Continuing Development of Priority Chronic Disease Indicators

- Continuing Development of Priority Maternal and Child Health Conditions and Events
- Control of Meningococcal Disease
- Coordination Between Federal and State Health Agencies of Outbreak Investigations Involving Products in Interstate Commerce
- Coordination of Surveillance Activities at CDC
- Cryptosporidium Contamination of Finished Water from Public Water Supplies
- CSTE Comments on USDA's Interim *Salmonella enteritidis* Regulations
- CSTE Support for the Guidelines for Coordination of Multistate Food-Borne Outbreak Investigations of the National Food Safety System Outbreak Coordination Work Group
- Data Sources for Surveillance of Vaccine-Preventable Diseases
- Decreasing the Spread of Antibiotic Resistance in the Community by Promoting More Judicious Antibiotic Use
- Defining Public Health Research and Public Health Nonresearch
- Definition for Case Surveillance of HIV Infection (Including AIDS)
- Definition of Public Health Research
- Deletions from the National Public Health Surveillance System
- Deterioration of the Capacity of the Centers for Disease Control and Prevention to Respond to Infectious Diseases
- Development of Environmental Public Health Indicators
- Development of Nationwide State-Based Chronic Disease Epidemiology Capacity
- Diagnosis and Treatment Guidelines for Infectious Diarrhea
- Diphtheria
- Discontinuation of Antimicrobials Used to Promote Growth of Food Animals if They Are Used in or Selected for Cross-Resistance to Antimicrobials Used in Human Therapy
- Disease Surveillance and Intervention Among American Indians and Alaska Natives
- *E. coli* 0157:H7
- Educational and Zoological Exhibits Which Allow Rabies Vector Human Contact
- Electronic Laboratory Reporting
- Electronic Laboratory Surveillance
- Emerging Infectious Diseases
- Encephalitis, Arboviral
- Encourage Federal Support for Vaccine Development Against Coccidioidomycosis
- Endorsement of Purpose and Methods of Surveillance Project

- Enhance National Effort to Contain or Eliminate Syphilis
- Enhancing Vaccine Delivery Infrastructure
- Environmental Health Capacity Building in State Health Agencies
- Environmental Health Competency Guidelines for State and Local Public Health Professionals
- Establishing a National Program for Venomous Snakebite Surveillance, Treatment, and Prevention
- Establishing an Oversight/Advisory Process for the Behavioral Risk Factor Surveillance System
- Establishment of a "No Year" Revolving Fund for Measles Outbreak Control
- Evaluation of the Impact of Vaccine Information Pamphlets on Immunization Levels
- Expanded Use of Hepatitis A Vaccine
- Extramural Funds for General Communicable Disease Activities
- Federal Expertise in Health Care Setting Ventilation Systems
- Firearm Injury and Deaths
- Folic Acid and the Prevention of Neural Tube Defects
- Funding for HIV/AIDS Surveillance
- Guidelines Regarding Cats and Rochalimaea Infection
- Head Injury Surveillance and Epidemiology
- Head Start Immunization Requirements
- Health and Risk Behavior Surveys of Youth
- Hepatitis, Viral, Perinatal Hepatitis B Virus Infection Acquired in the United States
- Hepatitis B Prenatal Screening Laws or Regulations
- Hepatitis B School and Child Day Care Entry Laws
- Hepatitis C Virus Infection (Chronic or Resolved)
- High-Priority Cancer Surveillance, Control, and Prevention
- HIV Home Collection Kits
- Human Parvovirus B19 and Pregnancy
- HUS Case Definition
- Immunization Amendment to the Employee Retirement Income Security Act of 1974
- Implementation of Integrated Communications Systems, Including Epidemic Information Exchange
- Implementation of Laboratory-Initiated CD4 Reporting Across All States
- Implementation of National Public Health Surveillance System (NPHSS)
- Implementation of the Pandemic Influenza Planning Guide for State and Local Health Officials

- Improved Laboratory Surveillance for HIV
- Improved Technology for Interagency Communication
- Improving Comparability of Chronic Disease Data Among the States
- Inclusion of Acute Pesticide-Related Illness and Injury Indicators in the National Public Health Surveillance System
- Inclusion of Acute Traumatic Brain Injury Indicators in the National Public Health Surveillance System
- Inclusion of Alcohol Use and Alcohol-Related Condition Indicators in the NPHSS
- Inclusion of Cancer Incidence and Mortality Indicators in the NPHSS
- Inclusion of Cancer Screening Indicators in the NPHSS
- Inclusion of Cardiovascular Disease Indicators in the NPHSS
- Inclusion of Childhood Dental Caries and Dental Sealants Indicators in the NPHHS
- Inclusion of Diabetes Surveillance Indicators in the NPHSS
- Inclusion of Drowning Indicators in the National Public Health Surveillance System
- Inclusion of End-Stage Renal Disease Indicators in the NPHSS
- Inclusion of Enterohemorrhagic *Escherichia coli* in the National Public Health Surveillance System (and Subsume *E. coli* O157:H7 Under EHEC).
- Inclusion of Firearm Injury Indicators in the National Public Health Surveillance System
- Inclusion of Fire Injury-Related Indicators in the National Public Health Surveillance System
- Inclusion of Intentional Injury Indicators in the National Public Health Surveillance System
- Inclusion of Motor Vehicle Injury-Related Indicators in the National Public Health Surveillance System
- Inclusion of Nutrition-Related Indicators in the NPHSS
- Inclusion of Oral Health Indicators in the NPHSS
- Inclusion of Osteoporosis-Related Conditions—Hip Fracture Indicators in the NPHSS
- Inclusion of Overarching Indicators of Health Status in the NPHSS
- Inclusion of Physical Inactivity Indicators in the NPHSS
- Inclusion of Poisoning Mortality and Morbidity in the National Public Health Surveillance System (NPHSS)
- Inclusion of Respiratory Disease Indicators in the NPHSS
- Inclusion of Selected Maternal and Child Health Conditions in the NPHSS

- Inclusion of Tobacco Surveillance Indicators in the NPHSS
- Inclusion of Varicella-Related Deaths in the NPHSS
- Inclusion of West Nile Encephalitis/Meningitis and Powassan Encephalitis/Meningitis in the National Public Health Surveillance System (NPHSS), and Revision of the National Surveillance Case Definition of Arboviral Diseases of the Central Nervous System (CNS)
- Increased CDC Focus on Chronic Disease Epidemiology in Both the EIS and the PMR
- Increased CSTE Focus on Chronic Disease Epidemiology
- Increasing Access to Sterile Syringes and Needles to Prevent Transmission of Blood—Federal Funding for West Nile Virus Surveillance, Research, and Control
- Indoor Use of Unvented Gas Heating and Cooking Appliances
- Infectious Diseases in Refugees
- Intensifying Surveillance and Reporting of Rubella Cases
- Intensifying Surveillance and Updating of Congenital Rubella Syndrome Case Definition
- Intradermal Rabies Vaccines
- Laboratory Screening for Antibiotic-Resistant *S. pneumoniae*
- Licensed Veterinarian
- Listeria Education for Pregnant Women
- Local-State-Federal Outbreak Investigation Coordination
- Maintenance of Nonhuman Primates As Pets
- Malaria
- Malaria Therapy Is Being Advocated by Some Physicians for Patients with Putative Lyme Disease
- Management of Contact Investigation for Tuberculosis Cases Who Travel on Commercial Airlines
- Meningococcal Disease Serogrouping and Vaccine Evaluation
- Meningococcal Vaccination
- Modification of Chronic Disease Indicators
- Modification of Medical Software and Aid Reporting
- More Timely National Death Reporting System
- National Goals for Adolescent Vaccination
- National HIV Surveillance: Addition to the National Public Health Surveillance System
- National Notification of Invasive Haemophilus Influenza Type b Disease
- The National Public Health Surveillance System
- National Public Health Surveillance System Recommendation—Survey of Tobacco Use

- National Reporting of Notifiable Diseases to Reflect Cases Reported by States and Territories
- National Surveillance for Cryptosporidiosis
- National Surveillance for Drug-Resistant *Streptococcus pneumoniae*
- National Surveillance for *Escherichia coli* O157:H7
- National Surveillance for Genital *Chlamydia trachomatis* Infections
- National Surveillance for Group A Streptococcal Invasive Disease
- National Surveillance for Hantavirus Disease
- National Surveillance for Hemolytic Uremic Syndrome
- National Surveillance of Drug Susceptibility Results of Isolates from Reported Tuberculosis
- National Surveillance of Invasive Group A Streptococcal Infection
- National Surveillance of Lyme Disease and Resources for Lyme Disease Epidemiology
- NCHS-State Data Coordination
- Need for Coordination of NEDSS, HAN, and Epi-X
- Notification of CDC Grant Awards to State Health Departments
- Occupational Disease Injury Surveillance
- Pediatric HIV Infection
- Pediatric HIV Infection Reporting
- Pertussis
- Placing Cyclosporiasis under National Surveillance in the United States
- Policy on Single-Project Assurances
- Prematriculation Immunization Requirements for Students Attending Colleges, Universities, and Other Institutions of Postsecondary School Education
- Prenatal Hepatitis B Screening
- Preschool Vaccination
- Prevention of Perinatal Transmission of HIV
- Proficiency of Rabies Testing Laboratories
- A Program to Develop Chronic Disease Epidemiologic Capacity at the State Level
- Promoting Adult Immunization Initiatives
- Promotion of Food Irradiation
- Proposal to Adopt Four New or Amended Surveillance Definitions for Environmental Health
- Psittacosis Surveillance Support
- Publication of Haemophilus Influenza Invasive Disease Data
- Public Health Activities for the Prevention and Control of Hepatitis C
- Public Health Response to Bioterrorism
- Public Health Response to Flooding in the United States

- Q Fever *(Coxiella burnetii)* Under National Surveillance in the United States
- Rabies Control
- Reciprocal (Interstate) Notification of HIV Cases
- Regional Surveillance for Coccidioidomycosis
- Reporting HIV and TB Comorbidity
- Reporting of Quarantinable Diseases
- Reporting of Traumatic Spinal Cord Injuries
- Reptile-Associated Salmonellosis and Prevention Education
- Restriction of Animal Rabies Vaccines to Use by or Under the Direct Supervision of a Licensed Veterinarian
- Review of Federal Regulations for the Shipment of Etiologic Agents and Clinical Specimens
- Review of the National Notifiable Disease Surveillance System (NNDSS)
- Revised Case Definitions for Public Health Surveillance: Infectious Disease
- Revised Case Definitions for Public Health Surveillance: Pertussis
- Revised Chronic Disease Indicators (CDI) to Reflect Expert and Stakeholder Recommendations
- Revised Surveillance Case Definition of HIV Infection
- Revision of Blood Lead Screening Recommendations and Regulations
- Revision of CDC Guidelines for Control of *Histoplasma capsulatum* and *Cryptococcus neoformans*
- Routine Drug Susceptibility Testing and Storage of MTB Isolates from Reported Tuberculosis Cases
- Rubella Syndrome, Congenital
- Securing Hepatitis A and Hepatitis B Vaccine for Adults at High Risk of Infection or the Serious Consequences of Infection
- Setting Priorities for Diseases, Conditions, and Health Status Indicators or Outcomes in the NPHSS
- Sexually Transmitted Diseases Screening and Surveillance in the United States
- Silicosis Surveillance and Case Definition
- Simplification and Unification of Immunization Schedules
- Specimen Submissions to NCID
- Standardizing the Structure of Public Health Case Definitions for Diseases and Conditions Placed Under the National Public Health Surveillance System
- Standards for Pediatric Immunization Practices
- Statement of Support for EPI-AID Investigations

- Statement on the Use of Nonculture Assays to Detect Communicable Infectious Agents
- Strengthening of State and Local Food-Borne Disease Prevention and Control Programs
- Strengthening the Nation's Public Health Defenses by Addressing Problems and Gaps in the Environmental Public Health System
- Support for Continued Evaluation of HIV/STD Prevention Program
- Support for Development and Implementation of the Epidemic Information Exchange
- Support for the Development of the National Action Agenda for Building Data Capacity for Maternal and Child Health
- Support of State-Based Efforts and Capacity for Translating Advances in Human Genetics into Public Health Action
- Support of State-Based Efforts and Capacity for Translating Advances in Human Responding to Citizen Concerns About Cancer and Cancer Clusters
- Surveillance and Control of Hepatitis B Virus Infection
- Surveillance Case Definition Changes
- Surveillance Case Definition for Adult Blood Lead Levels to Be Reported to the National Public Health Surveillance System
- Surveillance Definitions for Infections Occurring in Nonhospital Health Care Settings
- Surveillance for HBSAg-Positive Pregnant Women
- Surveillance for Hepatitis C
- Surveillance for HIV Incidence
- Surveillance for Invasive Pneumococcal Disease in Children Less than Five Years of Age
- Surveillance for Perinatal HIV Exposure
- Surveillance for STDs among Men Who Have Sex with Men
- Surveillance of Adolescent Tobacco Use
- Surveillance of HIV Infection and Disease
- Syphilis Control Strategies
- TB-HIV Surveillance and Control
- TB Prevention in Outpatient Health Care Settings
- Temporary Embargo on Importation of Cynomolgus Monkeys
- Training in Chronic Disease Programming
- Translocation of Wildlife
- Transport of Mosquito-Infested Vehicle Tires
- Tularemia As a Nationally Notifiable Disease
- Update "Statement on Ferrets" to Reflect New Scientific Data That Resulted in Changes in the National Recommendations on Rabies Exposure Management of Ferrets

- Use of Animal Rabies Vaccines for Species Not Specified on Label
- Use of Oxygenated Gasoline
- U.S.-Mexico Surveillance and Epidemiology Agreement
- Vaccine-Preventable Disease Surveillance and Reporting
- Validation of Data Representing Deaths Due to Vaccine-Preventable Diseases
- Varicella Surveillance and Control
- Visit for Adolescent Vaccinations and Other Preventive Health Issues

Emergency Nurses Association
<http://www.ena.org>

Position Statements

- Access to Health Care
- Advanced Practice in Emergency Nursing
- Approaching Diversity in Emergency Care
- Autonomous Emergency Nursing Practice
- Blood-Borne Infectious Diseases
- Care of Sexual Assault Victims
- Care of the Critically Ill or Injured Patient During Interfacility Transfer
- Care of the Pediatric Patient During Interfacility Transfer
- Chemical Impairment of Emergency Nurses
- Collaborative and Interdisciplinary Research
- Conscious Sedation
- Critical Incident Stress Management
- Customer Service in the Emergency Department
- Domestic Violence—Child Maltreatment and Human Neglect
- Educational Recommendations for Nurses Providing Pediatric Emergency Care
- Enhanced 9-1-1 Systems
- Family Presence at the Bedside During Invasive Procedures and/or Resuscitation
- Forensic Evidence Collection
- Hazardous Material Exposure
- Hospital and Emergency Department Overcrowding
- Injury Prevention
- Integration of Emergency Nursing Concepts in Nursing Curricula
- Latex Allergy
- Medical Evaluation of Suspected Intoxicated and Psychiatric Patients

- Minimal Trauma Nursing Education Recommendations
- Observation/Holding Areas
- The Obstetrical Patient in the Emergency Department
- Patients with Spontaneous Abortions in the Emergency Department
- Protection of Animal Subjects
- Protection of Human Subjects' Rights
- Resuscitative Decisions
- Role of Delegation by the Emergency Nurse in Clinical Practice Settings
- Role of the Emergency Nurse in Organ and Tissue Donation
- Role of the Registered Nurse in the Prehospital Environment
- Specialty Certification in Emergency Nursing
- Staffing and Productivity in the Emergency Care Setting
- Substance Abuse
- Telephone Advice
- Tuberculosis Exposure in the Emergency Department
- The Use of Non-Registered Nurse (Non-RN) Caregivers in Emergency Care
- The Use of the Newly Deceased Patient for Procedural Practice
- Violence in the Emergency Care Setting

Endocrine Society of Australia
<http://www.racp.edu.au/esa>

Position Statements
- Growth Hormone Replacement for Growth Hormone Deficiency in Adults, 1998
- Metaformin and Intervention in Polycystic Ovary Syndrome
- Use and Misuse of Androgens, 1999

European Society of Gene Therapy
<http://www.esgt.org>

Position Statement
- Strategic Issues for the Future of EU Gene and Cell Therapeutics

European Society of Human Genetics
<http://www.eshg.org>

Public Policy
- Data Storage and DNA Banking: Quality Issues, Confidentiality, Informed Consent
- Guidelines for the Provision of Genetic Services in Europe

- Insurance and Employment: Technical, Social, and Ethical Issues
- Screening: Technical and Ethical Issues, Including Commercialization of Genetic Tests

European Teratology Society
<http://www.etsoc.com>

Position Papers

- Male Fertility
- Statistical Analysis
- Vitamin A

Federation of American Societies for Experimental Biology
<http://www.fasdb.org>

Public Policy Priorities

- Animals in Research and Education
- Bioterrorism
- Cloning and Stem Cells
- Education and Professional Development
- Federal Funding
- Government Performance and Results Act
- Human Subjects in Research
- Indirect Costs
- Intellectual Property
- Medicare
- Priority Setting
- Public Service
- Regulatory Burden
- Research Integrity

Florida College of Emergency Physicians
<http://www.fcep.org/main.htm>

Position Statements

- The Baker Act
- Drowning Prevention
- Funding for EMRP
- Motorcycle Helmets

Genetics Society of America
<http://www.genetics-gsa.org>

Public Policy
- Evolution
- Genetically Modified Organisms

Georgia Academy of Family Physicians
<http://www.gafp.org>

Position Papers
- Access to Health Care
- Body Awareness for Adolescents
- Civil Justice Reform
- Cooperative Practice Between Family Physicians and Obstetricians in Maternity Care
- Georgia Health Care Reform
- Guidelines on the Supervision of Certified Nurse Midwives, Nurse Practitioners, and Physician Assistants
- HIV Infection/AIDS

Georgia Hospital Association
<http://www.gha.org/index.asp>

Position Statements
- Ambulatory Surgical Centers
- Medicaid Funding of Hospitals
- Nursing and Allied Health Shortages
- Patient Safety
- Timely Payment of Claims
- Tort Crisis
- Uninsured/Indigent Care

Healthcare Distribution Management Association
<http://www.healthcaredistribution.org>

Position Statements
- Continuous Availability of Prescription Medicines to the American Public
- Different Classes of Trade
- Electronic Compliance with Regulations
- Electronic Data Interchange
- Employee Testing and Monitoring

- Fair and Reasonable Drug Benefit Reimbursement
- FDA Patient Safety Initiative
- Free Enterprise Health Care System
- Medicare Prescription Drug Benefit
- Numerical and Automatic Identification of Health Care Products in Distribution and Patient Care
- Patient Privacy/Confidentiality of Health Care Records
- Pharmaceutical Therapy Management
- Recommended Identifier for E-commerce Transactions
- Returned Goods
- Right to Access
- State Licensure of Prescription Drug Distributors
- State Regulation of Third-Party Programs
- State Requirements for Controlled Substances and Precursor Chemicals
- Suggested Manufacturer Price Change Notification Policies and Procedures
- Suggested Pharmaceutical Manufacturer Product Shortage Policies and Procedures
- Warranty and Product Liability

Healthcare Information and Management Systems Society
<http://www.himss.org/asp/index.asp>

Hot Topics

- Bar Coding
- Clinical Informatics
- Data Mining
- E-commerce
- Financial Management
- National Preparedness and Response
- Patient Safety
- Privacy/Security/HIPAA
- Supply Chain Management

Health Industry Business Communications Council
<http://www.hibcc.org>

Position Statements

- Reduction of Medical Error
- 2-D Symbologies for Small Packaging Labeling

Health Physics Society
<http://www.hps.org>

Position Papers

- Background Information on "Ionizing Radiation—Safety Standards for the General Public"
- Background Information on "State and Federal Action Is Needed for Better Control of Orphan Sources"
- Clearance of Materials Having Surface or Internal Radioactivity
- Compatibility in Radiation-Safety Regulations
- Compensation for Diseases That Might Be Caused by Radiation Must Consider the Dose
- Food Irradiation
- Human Capital Crisis in Radiation Safety
- Ionizing Radiation—Safety Standards for the General Public
- Low-Level Radioactive Waste
- Occupational Radiation-Safety Standards and Regulations Are Sound
- Perspectives and Recommendations on Indoor Radon
- Radiation Risk in Perspective
- Risk Assessment
- State and Federal Action Is Needed for Better Control of Orphan Sources
- Ultraviolet Radiation and Public Health
- What About "Deadly Plutonium?"

Heart Rhythm Society
<http://www.hrsonline.org>

Position Statements

- Defibrillator Leads: Indications, Facilities, Training
- Recommendations for Extraction of Chronically Implanted Transvenous Pacing and the Role(s) of the Industry-Employed Allied Professional

Hospice and Palliative Nurses Association
<http://www.hpna.org>

Position Statement

- Legalization of Assisted Suicide

Hospital and Healthsystem Association of Pennsylvania
<http://www.haponline.org>

Position Statements
- Certificate of Need
- Degree-Granting Status of Hospital-Based Schools of Nursing and Allied Health
- Medicaid Fee-for-Service During Health Care Reform Transition
- Pooling Provisions of the Health Care Partnership Act

Illinois Hospital Association
<http://www.ihatoday.org>

Position Statements
- Disaster Readiness
- HIPAA
- Hospital Physician Relations
- KidCare
- Legal Issues
- Managed Care
- Medicaid
- Medicare
- Nursing
- Organ Donation
- Patient Safety
- Quality
- Telecommunications
- Uniform Billing Committee
- Uninsured

Illinois State Medical Society
<http://www.isms.org>

Professional Policies
- Abortion
- Abuse of Persons
- Access to Health Care
- Acupuncture
- Advertising Guidelines, Professional
- AIDS
- Alcoholism Education
- Alcoholism/Substance Abuse
- Ambulance Services

- Anaphylactic Reactions to Insect Stings
- Anatomical Gift Association of Illinois
- Animals in Research and Education
- Assessments
- Athletic Performance, Inappropriate
- Athletic Program
- Audits and Surveys
- Autopsies
- Birth Control
- Blood Availability
- Blood Services
- Breast Cancer Screening
- Child Safety Restraints
- Chronic Pain Patients
- Collective Bargaining
- Communication
- Confidentiality
- Conflict of Interest
- Continuing Education
- Corporate Practice of Medicine
- Cost Containment
- CPR
- Credentialing
- Current Procedure
- Death, Legal Definition
- Diabetes
- Diagnosis-Related Groups
- Dignity and Autonomy of Physicians
- Disaster Control
- Disclosure
- Discrimination Against Physicians
- DRG Payments and Cost of Procedures
- Drinking Age, Legal
- Driving Under the Influence
- Drug Formularies
- Drugs, Prescription
- Drug Use, Illegal
- Due Process
- Durable Power of Attorney
- Electromyoneurographic Procedures and Examinations
- Emergency Department Records
- Emergency Medical Care

- Entrepreneur Activity, Physician Ethics, Code of
- Ethics, Code of
- Euthanasia, Active Role of the Physician
- Executions, Physician Participation in
- Experimental Medical Procedures
- Expert Witness, Medical Testimony
- Eye Care
- Fees, Informing Patients of
- Freedom of Choice
- Freedom of Contract
- Handgun Control
- Health Care Costs
- Health Careers
- Health Care System Reform Principles
- Health Insurance, Voluntary Plans
- Health Maintenance Organizations
- Health Planning
- Health Screening by Allied Health Personnel
- Hearing Disorders
- Helmets
- Hospices
- Hospital and Medical Staff Committees
- Hospital Governing Boards
- Hospitalists, Opposition to Mandatory Use
- Hospital Medical Staff Management
- Hospital Medical Staff Privileges
- Human Cloning
- IDPA Drug Manual
- Immunization Programs
- Impaired Physicians
- Indemnification
- Indigent, Care of the
- Individual Rights
- Infant Feeding
- Infants Born with Disabilities
- Informed Consent
- Insanity As a Defense
- Insurance Companies, Collusion
- Joint Commission on Accreditation of Health Care Organizations
- Laboratories
- Legal Counsel
- Legislative Intrusion on Medical Judgment

- Managed Care
- Manipulative Casting of Congenital Deformities of the Extremities
- Marijuana
- Medical Diagnosis and Treatment
- Medical Education Schools
- Medical Examiners
- Medical Liability Insurance Premiums
- Medical Licensure
- Medical Psychotherapy
- Medical Representation in Government Planning
- Medical Staff As an Independent Organization
- Medical Staff Participation in Accreditation Activities
- Medical Staff Participation in Hospital Cost Containment Efforts
- Medical Staff Relationships with County Medical Society
- Medical Supplies, In-Flight
- Medical Testimony, Impartial
- Medicare Assignments
- Medicare Coverage
- Medicare Patients Contracting
- Membership
- Mental Health
- Multiphasic Screening
- National Health Insurance
- Newborns, Prenatal Development of
- Not-for-Profit Entities, Creating For-Profit Entities
- Nurse Practitioner
- Nurses' Education
- Nursing Homes
- Nutrition
- Occupational Health
- Optometric Services
- Organ Donor
- Patient Care Records and Their Availability
- Patient Discharge
- Patient Restraints
- Peer Review/Ethical Relations
- Physician/Patient Contract
- Physician/Patient Relationship
- Physician Profile, Access to
- Physician Records, Privacy of

- Physicians
- Physician's Assistants
- Preventive and Screening Services
- Primary Care
- Professional Associations
- Professional Liability
- Provider Organizations, Exclusive
- Public Aid
- Public Health Department
- Rehabilitation
- Reimbursement, Physician
- Reimbursement for Ambulatory Services
- Reimbursement for Outpatient Services
- Reimbursement for Treating Medicaid Patients
- Restrictive Covenants
- Risk Management
- Seat Belt Use
- Self-Referral/Physician Ownership
- Student Loans, Deductibility of Interest
- Surgery, Definition of
- Surgery, Laser
- Surgery, Psychosurgery
- Surgery, Reconstructive
- Surgery, Second Opinion
- Tanning Booths and Sunbeds
- Third-Party Intrusion into Medical Judgment
- Third-Party Payer Relationships
- Tobacco
- Unified AMA Membership
- Utilization Review
- Voluntary Health Organizations with Local Medical Communities
- Withdrawing or Withholding Life-Prolonging Treatment
- Workers' Compensation
- Workers' Right to Health Care

Infectious Diseases Society of America
<http://www.idsociety.org>

Position Statements

- Access to Clean Intravenous Injection Equipment
- Medicare Coverage of Outpatient Antimicrobial Therapy

Institute for Safe Medication Practices
<http://www.ismp.org>

Viewpoints
- Conceptual Framework for a National Medical Error Reporting Program
- Electronic Prescribing

Institute of Electrical and Electronics Engineers
<http://www.ieee.org/portal/site>

Position Statements
- Improving the Health Care System Through Use of Information Technologies
- Nondiscrimination in Employment Based on Genetic and Other Health Information
- Privacy, Confidentiality, and Security of Personal Health Information
- Quality of Health Information on the Internet
- U.S. Government Advisory Entities Concerned with Health-Related Issues

Intensive Care Society
<http://www.ics.ac.uk>

Position Statement
- Use of Activated Protein C

International and American Associations for Dental Research
<http://www.iadr.com>

Policy Statements
- Dietary Fluoride Supplements
- Fluoridation of Water Supplies

International Association of Orofacial Myology
<http://www.iaom.com>

Position Statements
- Diagnostic Label Tongue Thrust
- Nature and Evaluation of Oral Myofunctions

International Atherosclerosis Society
<http://www.athero.org>

Commentaries

- Advances in Neuroimaging of Acute Stroke
- Antioxidants and Cardiovascular Disease: Where Do We Stand?
- Cardioprotective Aspects of the Mediterranean and Japanese Diets
- The Danger of Drug Interactions in Antiatherosclerotic Therapy
- Dietary Fats
- Inflammation in Atherosclerosis—Causal or Casual?
- Mediterranean Diet, Olive Oil, and Cardiovascular Disease Incidence—The Case of Italy
- NCEP's ATP III Emphasizes the Metabolic Syndrome

International Commission on Occupational Health
<http://www.icoh.org.sg>

Position Statement

- Call for an International Ban on Asbestos

International Council of Nurses
<http://www.icn.ch>

Position Statements

- Abuse or Violence Against Nursing Personnel
- Acquired Immunodeficiency Syndrome
- Armed Conflict: Nurse's Perspective
- Assistive or Support Nursing Personnel
- Career Development in Nursing
- Child Labor
- Cloning and Human Health
- Distribution and Use of Breast Milk Substitutes
- Elimination of Female Genital Mutilation
- Elimination of Substance Abuse in Young People
- Ethical Nurse Recruitment
- Health Human Resources Development
- Health Information: Protecting Patient Rights
- Health Services for Migrants, Refugees, and Displaced Persons
- Impact of HIV/AIDS on Nursing/Midwifery Personnel
- Impact of the Use of High-Technology Equipment in Nursing Care
- International Trade Agreements
- Management of Nursing and Health Care Services
- Medical Waste: Role of Nurses and Nursing

- Mental Health
- Nature and Scope of Practice of Nurse-Midwives
- Nurse Retention, Transfer, and Migration
- Nurses and Disaster Preparedness
- Nurses and Human Rights
- Nurses and Primary Health Care
- Nurses and Shift Work
- Nurses and the Natural Environment
- Nurses' Role in Providing Care to Dying Patients and Their Families
- Nurses' Role in the Care of Prisoners and Detainees
- Nurses' Role in the Prevention and Early Detection of Cancer
- Nursing and Development
- Nursing Care of the Older Person
- Nursing Regulation
- Nursing Research
- Occupational Health and Safety for Nurses
- Participation of Nurses in Health Services Decision Making
- Part-Time Employment
- Patient Safety
- Prevention of Disability and the Care of People with Disabilities
- Promoting the Value and Cost-Effectiveness of Nursing
- Protection of the Title "Nurse"
- Reducing Environmental and Lifestyle-Related Health Hazards
- Reducing Travel-Related Communicable Disease Transmission
- Rights of Children
- Scope of Nursing Practice
- Socioeconomic Welfare of Nurses
- Strike Policy
- Tobacco Use and Health
- Torture, Death Penalty, and Participation by Nurses in Executions
- Toward Elimination of Weapons of War and Conflict
- Universal Access to Clean Water
- Women's Health

International Federation for the Surgery of Obesity
<http://www.obesity-online.com/ifso>

Position Statements

- Bariatric Surgeon Qualification
- Morbid Obesity and Its Treatment
- Patient Selection for Bariatric Surgery

International Federation of Environmental Health
<http://www.ifeh.org>

Policy Statements

- The Declaration of Kuala Lumpur
- The Declaration of Sydney
- Declaration on Environmental Health
- Environmental Health and Trade Agreements
- Environmental Health Management Systems
- Smoking
- Water and Sanitation

International Federation of Fertility Societies
<http://www.iffs-reproduction.org>

Consensus Statements

- Assisted Procreation
- Combination Oral Contraceptives and Cardiovascular Disease Surveillance
- Human Embryonic Stem Cells and Reproductive Cloning
- Tubal Infertility

International Federation of Sports Medicine
<http://www.fims.org/fims/frames.asp>

Position Statements

- AIDS and Sports
- Assessment of Subjects Older Than 35 Years
- Athletes with a Family History of Sudden Cardiac Death
- Bicycle Helmets
- Diabetes Mellitus and Exercise
- Doping
- Excessive Physical Training in Children and Adolescents
- Eye Injuries and Eye Protection in Sports
- Female Athlete Triad
- In-line Skating
- Scientific Commentary: Osteoporosis and Exercise
- Ventilatory Muscle Training in Patients with COPD

International Nurses Society on Addictions
<http://www.intnsa.org>

Position Papers

- Addictive Disorders Among Nurses and Nursing Students in Academic Settings
- AIDS
- Drug Testing
- Dual Diagnosis: A Model for Intermediate Care
- Educating Nurses on Addiction
- Outpatient Detoxification: Guidelines for Nurses
- Peer Assistance
- The Role of the Nurse in Alcoholism

International Occupational Hygiene Association
<http://www.ioha.com>

Policy Document

- Certification of Occupational Hygienists

International Osteoporosis Foundation
<http://www.osteofound.org>

Policy Initiatives

- A Call to Osteoporosis Action: European Union Policy Project/Consultation Panel
- European Community Initiatives on Osteoporosis
- IOF Position Statement on Milk Products and Osteoporosis
- Osteoporosis in the European Community: A Call to Action
- Recommendations from EU Report
- World Health Organization Strategy for Osteoporosis

International Pharmaceutical Foundation
<http://www.fip.org>

Position Statements

- Antimicrobial Resistance Control
- Counterfeit Medicines
- Electronic Prescriptions
- Genomics and Beyond
- Geriatric-Oriented Research
- Good Practice in Donating Medicines
- Good Practice in Pharmacy Education

- Labeling of Prescribed Medicines
- Medication Errors
- Paediatric-Oriented Research
- Pharmaceutical Care
- Pharmacist's Code of Ethics
- Product Selection
- Quality and Safety in Medicinal Products
- Responsible Self-Medication
- Self-Care Guidelines
- Teaching Children and Adolescents

International Society for Pharmacoepidemiology
<http://www.pharmacoepi.org>

Policy Statements
- Data Privacy, Medical Record Confidentiality, and Research in the Interest of Public Health
- Guidelines for Good Epidemiology Practices for Drug, Device, and Vaccine Research in the United States
- Power and Perils of Health Data Used in Epidemiologic and Economic Research

International Society of Nurses in Cancer Care
<http://www.isncc.org>

Position Statements
- Cancer Pain
- Cervical Screening
- Tobacco

International Society of Nurses in Genetics
<http://www.isong.org>

Position Statements
- Informed Decision Making and Consent: The Role of Nursing
- Privacy and Confidentiality of Genetic Information: The Role of the Nurse

International Society of Psychiatric-Mental Health Nurses
<http://www.ispn-psych.org>

Position Statements
- Alcohol Withdrawal Syndrome

- Clinical Psychologists with Prescriptive Authority
- Response to Clinical Psychologists Prescribing Psychotropic Medications
- Restraint and Seclusion
- Rights of Children in Treatment Settings
- White Paper on the Global Burden of Disease
- Youth Violence

Joint Council of Allergy, Asthma and Immunology
<http://www.jcaai.org>

Issues

- Compliance with Medicare Billing Rules for Allergy Immunotherapy
- Emergency Medical Treatment and Labor Act
- Insurance Coverage for H1-Antihistamines
- Medicare Payment

Juvenile Diabetes Research Foundation International
<http://www.jdf.org>

Policy Statements

- Diabetes Management in School
- Noninvasive and Minimally Invasive Blood Glucose Monitoring
- Stem Cell Research
- Strategic Research Plan of Diabetes Research Working Group
- Type 1 Diabetes and Vaccines
- U.S. Companies Discontinuing Production of Animal Insulin

Kansas Medical Society
<http://www.kmsonline.org>

Policy Resolutions

- Mandated Medical Screening Examinations
- Maternal and Infant Care
- Medical Records
- Patient-Physician Covenant
- Peer Review by State Disciplinary Agencies
- Physician Involvement in the Dying Process
- Physician-Patient Privilege
- Physician Responsibility and Cost Containment
- Smoking and Tobacco Product Sales
- Substance Abuse

Medical Society of New Jersey
<http://www.msnj.org>

Position Statements

- Abortion
- Biomedical Ethics
- Civil and Human Rights
- Drugs
- Environmental Health
- Health Care Delivery
- Health Care/System Reform
- Health Insurance
- HIV/AIDS
- Hospitals
- Legislation and Regulation
- Managed Care
- Maternal and Child Health
- Medical/Health Education
- Medicare
- Physician Fees
- Physicians
- Professional Liability
- Public Health
- Tobacco

Medical Society of the State of New York
<http://www.mssny.org/index.htm>

Position Statements

- Abortion and Reproductive Rights
- Accident Prevention
- Acquired Immunodeficiency Syndrome (AIDS)
- Alcohol and Alcoholism
- Alternative Health Care
- Children and Youth
- Chiropractic
- Clinical Judgment
- Computer Mailing Lists
- Continuing Medical Education
- County Medical Societies
- Death
- Drug Abuse

- Drug Dispensing
- Drugs and Medications
- Due Process for Physicians
- Education
- Environmental Health
- Ethics
- Family and Medical Leave
- Genetics
- Health Care Delivery Systems
- Health Care Professionals/Providers
- Health Insurance Coverage
- Health Screening Programs
- Health System Reform
- Home Health Care
- Homeless Shelters
- Hospice
- Hospitals
- Independent Practice of Medicine
- Licensure
- Managed Care
- Mandatory Medicaid Managed Care
- Medicaid
- Medical Data
- Medical Examiner System
- Medical Malpractice Panels
- Medicare
- Membership
- Mental Illness
- National Practitioner Data Bank
- Nuclear War, Weapons, and Terrorism
- Obstetrics
- Peer Review
- Physician Credentialing/Recredentialing
- Physician Discipline
- Practice Management
- Practice Parameters
- Professional Misconduct
- Protests and Demonstrations
- Public Health
- Reimbursement
- Rights and Responsibilities of Physicians
- Second Opinions and Consultations

- Second Opinions/Consultations—Terminology
- Sexual Harassment/Racial/Gender Discrimination
- Sports and Physical Fitness
- Surgery
- Tobacco Use and Smoking
- Universal Code for Reporting Medical Services
- Utilization Review
- Violence and Abuse
- Volunteer Services of Physicians
- Workers' Compensation

Michigan Society of Anesthesiologists
<http://www.mianesthesiologist.org>

Issues of Concern
- Terrorist Attacks

Midwives Alliance of North America
<http://www.mana.org>

Position Statements
- Access to Midwifery Care
- The Decriminalization of Midwifery
- Home Birth
- Intervention in Childbirth
- Midwifery Certification
- Midwifery Education
- The Midwifery Relationship with Women
- National Health Policy
- Policy Making and Resource Allocation
- Third-Party Reimbursement

Milwaukee Academy of Medicine
<http://dwp.bigplanet.com/academyofmed/door>

Position Statements
- Public Health and Education Committee Reports
- Public Health Strategies for Reducing Family and Intimate Violence
- Public Health Strategies to Reduce Alcohol-Related Illness, Injury, and Death
- Public Health Strategies to Reduce Tobacco-Related Illnesses and Deaths

Minnesota Medical Association
<http://www.mnmed.org>

Policy Statements

- Abortion
- Access to Health Care
- AIDS
- Alcohol/Alcoholism
- Allied Health Professionals
- Bicycle and Helmet Safety
- Birth Control
- Blood
- Board of Medical Practice
- Children and Youth
- Civil and Human Rights
- Civil Commitment
- Coding and Nomenclature
- Credentialing
- Data and Quality
- Death
- Domestic Violence and Abuse
- Driving While Intoxicated
- Elderly Persons
- Emergency Medical Care
- Environmental Health
- Ethics
- Fees
- Firearms
- Gambling
- Health Care Costs
- Health Care System Reform
- Health Education
- Health Fraud
- Hospitals
- Infection Control
- Laboratories
- Litigation
- Media
- Medical Education
- Medical Records
- Mental Health
- Minorities

- Motor Vehicle Safety
- Nursing Homes
- Organ Donation
- Peer Review
- Practice of Medicine
- Pregnancy
- Prescription Drugs
- Preventive Medicine
- Professional Liability
- Provider Contracting
- Public Health and Safety
- Public Programs
- Public Relations
- Reportable Diseases
- Research
- Rural Health and Underserved Areas
- Sports and Physical Fitness
- Support Services for Physicians
- Surgery
- Technology
- Third-Party Payers
- Tobacco
- Tort Reform
- Uninsured
- Utilization Review
- Veterans
- Violence
- Vital Statistics
- Vulnerable Adult Maltreatment
- Water Safety
- Workers' Comp

National Academy of Neuropsychology
<http://nanonline.org>

Position Papers
- Cognitive Rehabilitation
- Definition of a Neurophysiologist
- Technicians in Practice
- Test Security
- Third-Party Observers

National Association for Medical Direction of Respiratory Care
<http://www.namdrc.org>

Position Papers

- The Delivery of Hospital Respiratory Care
- Duties and Responsibilities of Medical Directors of Respiratory Care Services and Pulmonary Function Laboratories
- Respiratory Therapy: State Legal Credentialing
- Responsibilities of the Medical Director of the Pulmonary Physiology Laboratory
- State Respiratory Care Laws: Licensure Laws, Certification Laws, No Laws
- Ventilator Management

National Association of Community Health Centers
<http://www.nachc.com>

Issue Briefs

- Analysis of the Medicaid and Health-Related Provisions of the Personal Responsibility and Work Opportunity Reconciliation Act of 1996
- The Breast and Cervical Cancer Treatment and Prevention Act of 2000 (P.L. 106-354)
- Clarification of Health Center Employees, Including Clinicians, Discretion to Waive Patient Fees—Issue
- Clarification of the Balanced Budget Act's Policy Regarding Coverage of Emergency Services Under Medicaid Primary Care Case Management (PCCM)
- Contracting with a Pharmacy Management Service Company to Operate a Center's Licensed In-House Pharmacy
- DHHS, Office of the Inspector General's Special Advisory Bulletin Regarding the Prohibition of "Gainsharing" Arrangements and Civil Monetary Penalties for Hospital Payments to Physicians to Reduce or Limit Services to Beneficiaries: An Important Reminder on Medicare Site-by-Site Certification
- Enhancing Outreach and Enrollment Activities to Dual Eligibles in Health Centers
- Establishing a Cost-Based Charge Structure and Recording Patient Service
- Expanded Medicare Coverage of Diabetes Self-Management Training in Outpatient Settings

- Final Regulations on Standards for Privacy of Individually Identifiable Health Explanation of the Health Care Financing Administration's September 27, 2000, Letter to State Medicaid Directors Regarding Reimbursements to Federally Qualified Health Centers
- HCFA Issues New Guidance on Out Stationing That Strengthens Health Center Efforts at the State Level
- HCFA Medicaid Managed Care Guidance: Implementation of FQHC Balanced Budget Act Amendments
- HCFA's Policy Regarding Identification and Reinstatement of Medicaid Beneficiaries Whose Coverage Was Improperly Terminated As a Result of the 1996 Welfare Reform Law
- Health Centers Consolidation Act of 1996
- Immigrant Eligibility for Services at Health Centers
- Opportunities to Finance Health Professions Training Programs at Health Centers
- Oral Health and Access to Care: Eliminating Barriers for Low-Income Populations
- An Overview of Proposed Implementing Regulations for the State Child Health Insurance
- An Overview of Proposed Justice Department Regulations and Field Guidance Regarding Public Charge Determinations
- Program Fraud and Abuse
- Providing Health Care to Noncitizens: Summary and Overview of New HHS
- Safe Harbors for Shared Risk Arrangements
- Understanding a Health Center's Responsibility Regarding Collection of Medicare or Medicaid Copayments
- Understanding the Medicaid Prospective Payment System for Federally Qualified Health Centers
- The Volunteer Protection Act and Its Impact on Community Health Centers

National Association of Emergency Medical Technicians
<http://www.naemt.org>

Position Statements

- Access to Emergency Medical Services Act of 2001
- CONTOMS EMS Training Initiative
- Domestic Preparedness and Terrorism Response
- First Responder Terrorism Preparedness Act of 2002
- GSA KKK Specifications

- Hometown Heroes Survivors Benefits Acts of 2002
- National Center for Biomedical Research and Training Program Support
- Recommended Operational Security Measures
- Severe Acute Respiratory Syndrome
- Smallpox Vaccination

National Association of EMS Physicians
<http://www.naemsp.org>

Position Papers

- Acute Stroke: Implications for Prehospital Care
- Air Medical Dispatch: Guidelines for Scene Response
- Ambulance Diversion
- Clinical Guidelines for Delayed or Prolonged Transport I. Cardiorespiratory Arrest
- Clinical Guidelines for Delayed or Prolonged Transport IV. Wounds
- Criteria for Prehospital Air Medical Transport: Nontrauma and Pediatric Considerations
- Early Defibrillation Position Paper (January 2000)
- Emergency Medical Dispatching
- Emergency Medical Services and Emergency Medical Services Systems
- EMS Base Station Functional Design: Online Medical Control
- EMS Systems and Managed Care Integration
- Ethical Challenges in Emergency Medical Services
- Flight Physician Training Program
- Indications for Prehospital Spinal Immobilization
- Mass Gathering
- Medical Direction of Interfacility Transports
- Medical Director for Air Medical Transport Programs
- National Guidelines for Statewide Implementation of EMS "Do Not Resuscitate" Physician Medical Direction in EMS
- Prehospital Neuromuscular Blockade-Assisted Intubation
- Programs Prototype Curriculum for a Fellowship in Emergency Services
- Risk Reduction for Exposure to Blood-Borne Pathogens in EMS
- Role of EMS Physicians in EMS Education
- Special Resuscitation Issues Encountered During Air Medical Transport
- Subcutaneous Epinephrine for Out-of-Hospital Treatment of Anaphylaxis

- Sudden Cardiac Arrest and Early Defibrillation Position Statement (February 1998)
- Termination of Resuscitation in the Prehospital Setting for Adult Patients Suffering Nontraumatic Cardiac Arrest
- Use of Nitrous Oxide: Oxygen Mixtures in Prehospital Emergency Medical Care
- Use of the Pneumatic Antishock Garment (PASG)
- Use of Warning Lights and Sirens in Emergency Medical Vehicle Response and Patient Transport
- Verification of Endotracheal Tube Placement Following Intubation
- Voluntary Guidelines for Out-of-Hospital Practices

National Association of Neonatal Nurses
<http://www.nann.org/i4a/pages/index.cfm?pageid=1>

Position Statements and Resolutions

- Advanced Practice Neonatal Nurse Role
- BSN Entry into Practice
- Cobedding
- Cultural Competence
- Cup Feeding
- FNPs Being Used As NNPs
- Latex Allergy
- Minimum Staffing in NICUs
- Pain Management of Infants
- Scope of Practice for the Neonatal Staff Nurse
- Transport of Neonates Across State Lines
- Treatment of Critically Ill Newborns
- Use of Assistive Personnel in Providing Care to the High-Risk Infant

National Association of Nurse Practitioners in Women's Health
<http://www.npwh.org>

White Paper

- Quality Nurse Practitioner Education

National Association of Orthopaedic Nurses
<http://www.orthonurse.org>

Position Statements

- Adult Trauma
- Advanced Practice Nurses

- Blood-Borne Pathogens
- Health Care Reform
- Mandatory Seat Belt Legislation
- Osteoporosis As a National Public Health Priority in Health Care Reform
- Role of Unlicensed Assistive Personnel in Orthopedic Nursing Care

National Association of Pediatric Nurse Practitioners
<http://www.napnap.org/index_home.cfm>

Philosophical Statements

- Children
- Continuing Education
- Health

Position Statements

- Breast-feeding
- Certification for Advanced Nursing Practice
- Child Abuse/Neglect
- Child Care
- Corporal Punishment
- Entry into Practice
- Health Care Reform for Children
- Health Risks and Needs of Gay, Lesbian, Bisexual, and Transgender Adolescents
- Immunization
- Mandatory HIV Testing in Health Care Workers
- Newborn Discharge and Follow-up Care
- Pediatric HIV Disease
- Prevention of Tobacco Use in the Pediatric Population
- School-Based and School-Linked Clinics
- Third-Party Payment

National Association of Public Hospitals and Health Systems
<http://www.naph.org>

Issues Advocacy

- Access to Care for the Uninsured
- Community Access Program
- EMTALA
- Immigration
- Medicaid
- Medicaid DSH

- Medicaid Upper Payment Limits
- Medicare DSH
- Medicare Outpatient Prospective Payment System
- Medicare Reform
- State Children's Health Insurance Program
- Workforce

National Association of School Nurses
<http://www.nasn.org>

Position Statements

- Adolescent Parents
- Advanced Practice School Nurse
- Asthma Inhalers
- Automatic External Defibrillators in the School Setting
- Caseload Assignments
- Case Management
- Child Abuse and Neglect
- Child Care
- Condom Availability in the School Setting
- Continuing Education
- Contract Provisions
- Coordinated School Health Program
- Corporal Punishment
- Delegation
- Do Not Resuscitate
- Emergency Care Plans for Students with Special Health Care Needs
- Family Life Education
- Government Relations: Public Policy, Legislative, and Regulatory Participation
- Hazing
- Healthy School Environment
- Immunizations
- Individualized Health Care Plans
- Indoor Air Quality
- Infectious Disease
- Managed Care
- Medication Administration in the School Setting
- Mental Health of Students
- Natural Rubber Latex Allergy
- Nit-Free Policies in the Management of Pediculosis
- Nursing Diagnosis

- Nursing Minimum Data Set for School Nursing Practice
- Out-of-School Education: Field Trips and Camps
- Postural Screening
- Professional School Nurse Roles and Responsibilities: Education, Certification, and Licensure
- Reduction in Force
- Regulations on Blood-Borne Pathogens in the School Setting
- Role of the School Nurse in Violence Prevention
- School-Based/School-Linked Health Centers
- School Health Records
- School Meal Programs
- School Nurse and Specialized Health Care Services
- The School Nurse and Sun Protection
- School Nurse Attire
- School Nurse in Comprehensive School Health Education
- School Nurse Practitioners
- School Nurse Supervision/Evaluation
- Sexual Orientation
- State School Nurse Consultants
- Substance Use and Abuse
- Volunteers in the Health Office
- Wellness Programs

Issue Briefs

- Delegation of Care
- Health Care Reform and Schools
- Inclusion
- Integrated Service Delivery
- Managed Care
- Mental Health and Illness
- School-Based/School-Linked Clinics
- School Nurses and the Individuals with Disabilities Act
- School Violence

National Association of School Psychologists
<http://www.nasponline.org>

Position Statements

- Ability Grouping
- Advocacy for Appropriate Educational Services for All Children
- Assessment, School Psychologists' Involvement in the Role of
- Assessment Experts

- Attention Problems
- Comprehensive Service Delivery
- Corporal Punishment in Schools
- Early Childhood Assessment
- Early Childhood Care and Education
- Early Intervention Services
- Effective Parenting: Positive Support for Families
- Emotional and Behavioral Disorders
- Gay, Lesbian, and Bisexual Youth
- HIV/AIDS
- Home-School Collaboration
- Inclusive Programs for Students with Disabilities
- Interagency Collaboration to Support the Mental Health Needs of Children and Families
- Mental Health Services in the Schools
- Minority Recruitment
- Pupil Services: Essential to Education
- Racism, Prejudice, and Discrimination
- Rights Without Labels
- School Violence
- Sexuality
- Student Grade Retention and Social Promotion
- Three-Year Reevaluations for Students with Disabilities

National Community Pharmacists Association
<http://www.ncpanet.org>

Position Statements

- Alternative Health Care Delivery Systems
- Alternative Prescription Distribution
- Arbitrary Changing of AWP
- Assisted-Living Facility Regulations
- Certification and Accreditation
- Color Coding of Pharmaceuticals by Strength
- Compounding by Pharmacists
- Consumer Freedom of Choice
- Consumer Right-to-Know Participating Pharmacies
- Co-op Buying
- Current Drug Information
- DEA and Health Care Professionals
- Direct-to-Consumer Advertising
- Direct-to-Patient Health Care Information

- Discriminatory Pricing Policies
- Diversion of Prescription Drugs
- Drug Benefit Equity
- Drug Look-Alikes
- Drug Recalls
- Earned Discounts
- Electronic Prescribing and Data Transmissions
- Employee Retirement Income Security Act (ERISA)
- Entrepreneurship and Free Enterprise
- Equal Access
- Equal Access to Cost Containment Strategies
- Equitable Pricing
- Expiration Dates
- FDA Approval Labeling
- FTC Interference and Inaction
- Generic Drug Dispensing Incentives
- Health Insurance Portability and Accountability Act (HIPAA)
- Home Health Care
- Homeopathy
- Hospital Outpatient Dispensing
- Indemnity Insurance Prescription Plans
- Insurance Antitrust Reform
- Internet Pharmacies
- Interprofessional Relations
- Joint Commission of Pharmacy Practitioners
- Joint Commission on Accreditation of Healthcare Organizations
- Long-Term Care Accreditation
- Long-Term Care and Managed Care
- Long-Term Care Drug Therapy
- Long-Term Care Pharmacy and Fair Trade Mail Order Sales Taxes
- Managed Care Improvement
- Marketplace Pricing
- MedGuide
- Medicaid Outpatient Drug Program
- Medical Savings Accounts
- Medicare Billing for DME Drugs
- Medicare Reform: JCPP Statement
- Narrow Therapeutic Index Medications
- Nationwide Prescriber Identification Number System
- NDC Numbers
- New USP Environmental Standards
- Patient Confidentiality

- Patient Counseling
- Patient Package Inserts
- Patients' Bill of Rights
- P.D. Designation
- Pharmacist Care
- Pharmacist Consultation on OTC Labeling
- Pharmacist Legend
- Pharmacy Benefits Information for Consumers
- Pharmacy Benefits Manager (PBM) Discounts
- Pharmacy Benefits Manager (PBM) Formularies
- Pharmacy Benefits Manager (PBM) Oversight
- Pharmacy Entry-Level Degree
- Pharmacy Participation in Federal Programs
- Pharmacy Services for All Americans
- Pharmacy Student Entrepreneurial Programs
- Pharmacy Technicians
- Physician and Pharmacist Cooperation
- Physician Drug and Device Sales for Profit
- Physician Extenders
- Polygraph Testing
- Prescription Benefit Identification Cards
- Price Controls
- Price Increases Notification
- Professional Services Payment
- Prospective Payment System
- Recognition of Pharmacists As Health Care Providers
- Restricted Distribution of Pharmaceuticals
- Returned Goods Policies
- Robinson-Patman Act
- Sampling of Prescription Drugs
- Selection of Government Health Officials
- Small Business Health Insurance Tax Equity
- Starter Doses, Bonus Products, and Indigent Patient Programs
- Tamper-Resistant Packaging
- Technician Support and Technology
- Third-Party Administrator Regulation
- Third-Party Claims Transmission Costs
- Third-Party Contract Quality Pharmacist Care
- Third-Party Negotiations
- Third-Party Price Updates
- Third-Party Program Decision Making

- Tobacco Sales
- Unfair Reimbursement Rates in Home Health Care
- United States Pharmacopoeia
- Unregulated Mail Order Drug Programs
- Vendor Access to Government-Supported Health Programs
- Veterans' Freedom of Choice
- Veterinary Drugs

National Council of State Boards of Nursing
<http://www.ncsbn.org>

Position Statement
- Foreign Nurse Immigration

National Dental Association
<http://www.ndaonline.org>

Position Statements
- Health Care Reform
- Managed Care

National Environmental Health Association
<http://www.neha.org>

Position Statements and Resolutions
- Antibiotic Feed and Human Health
- Children's Environmental Health
- Endocrine Disrupters
- Global Climate Change
- Pesticides
- Resolution of Secondhand Tobacco Smoke
- Resolution Regarding Community Water Fluoridation
- Resolution Regarding Genetically Modified Organisms
- Resolution to Support a Federal Trade Commission Requirement for Surgeon General Warning Labels on Cigars
- Resolution to Support a Global Approach to the Prevention of Youth Tobacco Use
- Resolution to Support Public Health Principles and Guidance for Brownfields Policies and Practices
- Resolution to Support the Clean Air Act Amendments
- Resolution to Support the Responsible Irradiation of Foods

National Family Planning and Reproductive Health Association
<http://www.nfprha.org>

Position Statement
- Women's Right to Know

National Health Council
<http://www.nationalhealthcouncil.org>

Position Papers
- Direct-to-Consumer Pharmaceutical Advertising
- Discriminatory Practices Based on Medical Information
- Human Cloning and Cloning Legislation
- Medical Records Privacy
- Medicare Coverage of Prescription Drugs
- Stem Cell Research

National Rural Health Association
<http://www.nrharural.org>

Issue Papers
- Access to Health Care for the Uninsured in Rural and Frontier America
- Antitrust and Rural Health
- Community Health Advisor Programs
- Essential Community (Access) Providers
- Facilitating the Use of National Surveys in Rural Health Research
- Funding of Graduate Medical Education
- HIV/AIDS in Rural America
- The Impact of Entitlement Programs on Rural Health
- Managed Care As a Delivery Model in Rural Areas
- Mental Health in Rural America
- A National Agenda for Rural Minority Health
- The Need for a National Limited-Service Hospital Program
- The Role of Telemedicine in Rural Health Care
- Rural and Frontier Emergency Medical Services Toward the Year 2000
- Rural Health Clinics in Rural America
- Rural Physician Recruitment and Retention
- A Vision for Health Reform Models for America's Rural Communities

National Society of Genetic Counselors
<http://www.nsgc.org>

Position Statements

- Access to Care
- Confidentiality of Test Results
- Cystic Fibrosis
- Disclosure and Informed Consent
- DNA Sequencing Position Statement
- Fetal Tissue Research
- Genetic Screening
- Genetic Testing and Adoption Position Statement
- National Health Care Reform
- Nondiscrimination
- Prenatal and Childhood Testing for Adult-Onset Disorders
- Prenatal Substance Abuse
- Reproductive Freedom

New Hampshire Hospital Association
<http://www.nhha.org/index-nhha.php>

Policy Statements

- Access to Care
- Appropriate Levels of Care
- Certificate of Need
- Civil Liability and Tort Reform
- Collaboration and Competition
- Communicable Diseases
- Community Benefit
- Community Care Networks
- Confidentiality
- Consent
- Data Collection and Disclosure
- End-of-Life Care
- Environmental Protection
- Essential Community Providers
- Gender Equity
- Governance
- Health Promotion
- Organ and Tissue Donation
- Patient Safety and Quality

- Payment Systems
- Professional Licensure and Certification
- Provider-Sponsored Networks
- Tax Status
- Workforce

New Hampshire Public Health Association
<http://www.nhpha.org>

Policy Statements
- Access to Care
- Alcohol and Other Drugs
- Child Health and Safety
- Elderly
- Environmental Health
- Food Safety
- Health Education and Promotion
- HIV/AIDS
- Infectious Diseases
- Managed Care
- Occupational Health
- Oral Health
- Reproductive Health
- Smoking
- Unintentional Injury
- Violence

Ontario Medical Association
<http://www.oma.org>

Position Papers
- Secondhand smoke
- Timely Return to Work
- Tobacco

Ontario Orthopaedic Association
<http://www.ooa.on.ca>

Position Paper
- Patient Access to Orthopedic Surgical Care

Oregon Association of Hospitals and Health Systems
<http://www.oahhs.org>

Topical Issues

- AHA Quality Advisory IOM Report on Medication Errors
- AHA's Medicare Outpatient PPS Regulatory Alert
- Assessing the Financial Impact of Outpatient PPS
- Balanced Budget Relief Act Legislation
- BIPA Legislation Summary
- Federal Poverty Guidelines
- Final PPS Regulations Published
- HCFA Guidelines on Patient Dumping
- I.S. Security versus Privacy—Essentials of a Privacy Policy
- President's Proposal on Medical Errors
- Prospective Payment System for Hospital Outpatient Services
- Recovering Lost Revenue

Pharmaceutical Care Management Association
<http://www.pcmanet.org>

Policy Statements

- Confidentiality of Patient Identifiable Health Information
- Consumer Access to Affordable Pharmaceutical Benefits
- Licensure of Pharmacy Benefit Managers
- Mail Service Pharmacy Regulation
- Medicare Prescription Drug Coverage
- Plan-Sponsored Drug Formularies and Formulary Management

Pharmaceutical Society of Australia
<http://www.psa.org.au>

Position Statements

- Complementary Medicines
- Coordinated Care
- Distance Dispensing
- National Medicinal Drug Policy
- Pharmaceutical Benefits Scheme
- Pharmaceutical Care
- Schedule 3 Advertising
- Therapeutic Group Premiums

Public Health Association of Australia
<http://www.phaa.net.au>

Policy Statements
- Aboriginal and Torres Strait Island Health
- Child Health
- Disease Prevention
- Drugs
- Environmental Health
- Food and Health
- Health Care Financing
- Health Services Development
- Housing
- Immunization
- Infectious and Transmittable Diseases
- Information and Health Statistics
- Injury
- International Health and International Trade
- Lifestyle Choices
- Mental Health
- Political Economy of Health
- Population Health
- Reproductive Health
- Research
- Weapons and War
- Women's Health
- Workforce Training and Development
- Youth Health

Public Health Association of New York City
<http://www.phanyc.org>

Policy Statements
- "Competition," Premium Support Proposals, and Prescription Drug Benefits Under Medicare
- Making Medicines Affordable: The Price Factor

Respiratory Nursing Society
<http://www.respiratorynursingsociety.org>

Position Statements
- Development of Nonchlorofluorocarbon Metered-Dose Inhalers
- Long-Term Oxygen Therapy

Royal Australasian College of Physicians
<http://www.racp.edu.au>

Health and Social Policy

- Breast-feeding
- Circumcision
- Compensable Injuries and Health Outcomes
- Ethics of Research in Children
- Examination of the Newborn
- For Richer, for Poorer, in Sickness and in Health: The Socioeconomic Determinants of Health
- From Hope to Science: Illicit Drugs Policy in Australia
- Getting in the Picture: Guide for the Better Use of Television for Children
- Guidelines for the Funding of Paediatric Research by Formula Companies
- Human Milk Banking
- Indigenous Health Education and Resource Guide
- Paediatrician Attendance at Caesarean Sections
- Paediatric Policy
- Physical Punishment and Discipline (Including Smacking)
- Protecting Children Is Everybody's Business
- Protecting Children Is Everybody's Business: Paediatricians Responding to the Challenge of Child Abuse
- Reducing Blood Lead Levels in Australian Children
- Soy Protein Formula
- Submission to the Working Party: The Use of Cannabis for Medicinal Purposes
- Vitamin K
- Vitamin K for Newborn Babies: Information for Parents

Royal Australasian College of Surgeons
<http://www.surgeons.org>

Nontechnical Policy Statements

- Aboriginal and Torres Strait Islander Health Organization
- Advertising
- Appeals Mechanism
- Entrepreneurial Aspects of Medical Practice
- Ethics
- FRACS Suffix and Descriptors
- Media

- Medical Records
- Multiple Housing Appointments
- Operating on Family Members
- Payment of Fellows
- Private Health Insurance
- Private Hospitals on Public Campuses
- Publications
- Public Patients in Private Hospitals
- Public Relations
- RACS Representatives on Hospital Electoral Bodies
- Retirement Age
- Review of Standards of Practice for Outside Organizations
- Rewarding Excellence in Surgery
- Waiting Lists for Elective Surgery

Technical Policy Statements

- Accreditation of Surgical Services in Hospitals
- Auditing of Breast Cancer Surgical Procedures
- Autologous Blood Transfusion in Elective Surgery
- Boxing
- Chiropractic
- Credentialing Processes—New Technology and Surgical Practice
- Credentials Committees—Guidelines for Fellows Action As College Spokesman on Credentials Committees
- Delineation of Responsibilities
- Disciplinary Procedures
- Endoscopy
- Extracorporeal Perfusion
- Female Genital Mutilation
- General Practitioners and Surgery
- Gun Control
- Impaired Surgeon
- Infection Control in Surgery
- Itinerant Surgery
- Laparoscopic Cholecystectomy
- Male Circumcision
- Mammography
- Multidisciplinary Management of Paediatric Tumors
- New Technology and Surgical Practice
- Operating with Open Wounds for Dermatitis on the Hands
- Oral and Maxillofacial Surgery
- Paediatric Surgery

- Podiatry
- Policies Incorporating the Implications of New Technology for Surgical Practice, Quality Assurance, Accreditation, and the Delineation of Responsibilities
- Prostheses and Implants
- Quality Assurance and Manpower Policy Statements
- Quality Assurance/Clinical Indicators
- Recertification
- Relations with Dermatologists
- Rural Surgery
- Sedation for Endoscopy
- Smoking
- Standards of Surgical Services in Hospitals and Their Assessment
- Surgical Assistants
- Surgical Audit
- Tattoos
- Transplantation
- Trauma and Road Trauma

Royal Australian and New Zealand College of Psychiatrists
<http://www.ranzcp.org>

Position Statements

- Abolition of Torture
- Alcohol Misuse and Dependence
- Continuing Medical Education Within the College
- Deep Sleep Therapy
- Firearm Legislation in Australia
- HIV/AIDS
- Methadone Prescription by Psychiatrists
- Orthomolecular Psychiatry
- Pathological/Problem Gambling
- Policy on Mental Health Services
- Position Statement on Psychosurgery
- Principles on the Provision of Mental Health Services to Asylum Seekers
- Psychiatry Services for the Elderly
- Recent Changes to Australian National Mental Health Policy
- Relationships Between Geriatric and Psychogeriatric Services
- The Role of Psychiatrists in Disasters
- The Safe Use of Clozapine
- St. John's Wort

- Stolen Generations
- Telepsychiatry
- Transcranial Magnetic Stimulation
- What Is a Psychiatrist? What Does a Psychiatrist Do?

Royal Australian and New Zealand College of Radiologists
<http://www.racr.edu.au/index.htm>

Policy Statements

- Breast Imaging
- Contrast
- CT
- Faculty of Radiation Oncology Quality Assurance
- Medical Imaging
- Radiotherapy in Rural Australia
- Teleradiology
- Ultrasound

Royal Australian College of General Practitioners
<http://www.racgp.org.au>

Position Statements

- Aboriginal Health
- After-Hours Primary Medical Care in General Practice
- Co-coordinated Care
- The Context of General Practice
- Definition of General Practice
- Domestic Violence
- Evidence-Based Medicine (EBM)
- General Practice Management
- Health and the Environment
- Health Issues and Issues of Service Delivery
- Hepatitis B Immunization
- Immunization
- Information Management and the Role of Information Technology
- Joint Statement on Pap Smears
- Nurse Practitioners
- Prevention and Health Promotion in General Practice
- Quality Assurance and Continuing Education
- The RACGP and the Profession
- The RACGP Research Program
- The RACGP Training Program

- Relationships Between General Practice and Community Health
- The Role of GPs in Relation to Hepatitis C Virus Infection
- The Roles of GPs in Relation to HIV Infection
- The Role of GPs in the Delivery of Health Care to Women
- The Role of GPs in the Delivery of Mental Heath Services
- The Role of GPs in the Provision of Health Care for Older Persons
- Roles of the College
- Standards in General Practice
- Vision for the College
- Vision Statement for General Practice
- Youth Suicide

Royal College of General Practitioners
<http://www.rcgp.org.uk>

Position Statements

- Clinical Governance in Primary Care—Practical Advice on Implementation
- Confidentiality—Examining the Principle of Medical Confidentiality
- Domestic Violence: The General Practitioner's Role
- Implementing a Scheme for GPs with Special Clinical Interests
- Primary Care and Local Health Groups: Risks, Opportunities, and the Way Forward
- The Primary Care Workforce—An Update for the New Millennium
- Removal of Patients from GPs' Lists: Guidance for College Members

Policy Documents

- Education and Training for General Practice
- Evidence to the Royal Commission on the National Health Service
- Quality in General Practice

Discussion Documents

- Access to General Practice-Based Primary Care
- The Future of Professionally Led Regulation for General Practice
- Is There a Future for Independent Contractor Status in UK General Practice?

Royal College of Nursing
<http://www.rcn.org.uk>

Policy Initiatives

- Equality Issues
- Partnership Working
- Political Devolution
- Prescribing
- UK Nursing Strategies

Royal College of Nursing (Australia)
<http://www.rcna.org.au>

Position Statements

- Advanced-Practice Nursing
- Community Immunization—Children/Adolescent
- Complementary Therapies in Australian Nursing Practice
- Conscientious Objection
- Continuing Professional Development
- Enrolled Nurse
- Ethics in Nursing Practice
- Health Promotion
- Health Services for Aboriginal and Torres Strait Islander People
- Joint Position Statements on Unregulated Workers and Nursing Care
- Management of Nursing and Midwifery Services
- Nurses, Health, and the Environment
- Nursing Education for Aboriginal and Torres Strait Island People
- Nursing Practice in a Culturally Diverse Australian Society
- Nursing Practice in Relation to Blood-Borne Viral Infections
- Nursing Research
- Primary Health Care
- Quality in Nursing Practice
- Registered Nurses and the Quality Use of Medicine
- Registered Nurses in Aged Care Facilities and Quality Use of Medicines
- The Role of Nurses in Palliative Care
- The Role of Nurses in the Management of Cardiorespiratory Arrest
- Smoking and Health
- Social Policy and Health
- Voluntary Euthanasia/Assisted Suicide

Royal College of Obstetricians and Gynaecologists
<http://www.rcog.org.uk>

Guideline Summaries

- The Care of Women Requesting Induced Abortion
- The Initial Investigation and Management of the Infertile Couple
- The Initial Management of Menorrhagia
- Male and Female Sterilisation
- The Management of Infertility in Secondary Care
- The Management of Infertility in Tertiary Care
- The Management of Menorrhagia in Secondary Care

Working Party Reports

- Clinical Governance
- Intimate Examinations
- Maintaining Good Medical Practice
- Management of Vulval Cancer
- Revalidation
- Standards in Colposcopy
- Storage of Ovarian and Prepubertal Testicular Tissue
- Toward Safer Childbirth
- Ultrasound Screening

Study Group Recommendations

- Disorders of the Menstrual Cycle
- Evidence-Based Fertility Treatment
- Fetal Programming—Influences on Development and Disease in Later Life
- Gene Identification, Manipulation, and Therapy
- Hormones and Cancer
- The Placenta: Basic Science and Clinical Practice
- Prevention of Pelvic Infection
- Problems in Early Pregnancy
- Screening for Down Syndrome in the First Trimester
- Violence Against Women

Royal College of Pathologists of Australasia
<http://www.rcpa.edu.au/public/default.cfm>

Policy Statements

- Automated and Semiautomated Cervical Screening Devices
- Autopsies and the Use of Tissue Removed at Autopsy
- Complaints Handling

- Ethical Responsibility of Pathologists in Relation to Test Utility
- Histological Review of Tissue Removed from Patients
- Items and Services Pathologists May Provide in the Collection of Pathology Samples
- Laboratory Categorisation
- Nurse Practitioners and Pathology Test Ordering
- Provision of Second Opinions
- Routine Rescreening of Gynaecological Cytology
- Specimens
- Surgical Specimen Cut Up
- Telepathology

Royal College of Physicians and Surgeons of Canada
<http://rcpsc.medical.org/index.php?pass=1>

Policy Statements and Guidelines

- Acquisition Policy for Books and Monographs for the Roddick Room Collection
- Criteria for Recognition of a Subspecialty for Purposes of Accreditation of a Residency Program
- Guidelines for RCPSC Academic Certification
- Guidelines for Support of Continuing Medical Education by Industry
- Policy on Conflict of Financial Interest
- Policy Regarding Publication of RCPSC Qualifications/Specialties Recognized by the RCPSC

Royal College of Physicians of London
<http://www.rcplondon.ac.uk>

Working Party Reports

- Acute Medicine: The Physician's Role
- ALCOHOL—Can the NHS Afford It?
- The Cancer Patient's Physician
- Cancer Units—Improving Quality in Cancer Care
- The Health and Care of Older People in Care Homes
- Management of the Older Medical Patient
- Medical Rehabilitation
- Nicotine Addiction in Britain
- Prescribing Costly Medicines
- Principles of Pain Control in Palliative Care for Adults
- Skill Mix and the Hospital Doctor

- Training in Academic Medicine
- Women in Medicine

Royal College of Psychiatrists
<http://www.rcpsych.ac.uk>

Council Reports

- Alcohol and the Heart in Perspective
- Assessment and Clinical Management of Risk of Harm to Other People
- The Association Between Antipsychotic Drugs and Sudden Death
- Behavioural and Cognitive Treatments
- Benzodiazepines: Risks, Benefits, or Dependence—a Reevaluation
- Care of Older People with Mental Illness
- Chronic Fatigue Syndrome
- Clinical Practice Guidelines and Their Development
- College Statement on Rape
- Community Care
- Consensus Statement on the Assessment and Investigation of an Elderly Person with Suspected Cognitive Impairment by a Specialist Old Age Psychiatry Service
- Consensus Statement on the Use of High-Dose Antipsychotic Medication
- Curriculum for Basic Specialist Training and the MRCPsych Examination
- Development of Psychological Therapy Services: Role of the Consultant Psychotherapist
- Eating Disorders in the UK: Policies for Service Development and Training
- Ethical Issues in Psychiatric Practice in Prisons
- Gender Identity Disorders in Children and Adolescents: Guidance for Management
- The General Hospital Management of Adult Deliberate Self-Harm
- Good Medical Practice in the Psychiatric Care of Potentially Violent Patients in the Community
- Good Psychiatric Practice
- Good Psychiatric Practice—Confidentiality
- Guidance for Researchers and for Ethics Committees on Psychiatric Research Involving Human Participants
- Guidance for the Use of Video Recording in Child Psychiatric Practice
- Guidance for Videotaping

- Guidance on Staffing for Child and Adolescent Inpatient Psychiatric Units
- Guidelines for Health Care Commissioners for an ECT Service
- Homelessness and Mental Illness
- Institutional Abuse of Older Adults
- Managing Deliberate Self-Harm in Young People
- Meeting the Mental Health Needs of People with Learning Disability
- Mental illness: Stigmatization and Discrimination Within the Medical Profession
- Offenders with Personality Disorder
- Organophosphate Sheep Dip: Clinical Aspects of Long-Term Low-Dose Exposure
- Patient Advocacy
- Perinatal Maternal Mental Health Services: Recommendations for Provision of Services for Childbearing Women
- Policy for Patients' Monies
- Prevention in Psychiatry
- Psychiatric Rehabilitation
- Psychiatric Services for Children and Adolescents with Learning Disabilities
- Psychiatric Services to Accident and Emergency Departments
- Psychological Therapies for Adults in the NHS: A Joint Statement by the British Psychological Report on the Position of Psychiatry in the Republic of Ireland
- Reciprocity Between the Royal College of Psychiatrists and the Royal Australian and New Zealand College of Psychiatrists
- Report of the Ethnic Issues Project Group
- Report of the Overseas Working Group
- Report of the Working Group on Standards of Places of Safety Under Section 136 of the Mental Health Act (1983)
- Report of the Working Group on the Size, Staffing, Structure, Siting, and Security of New Acute Adult Psychiatric Inpatient Units
- Report of the Working Party on the Psychological Care of Surgical Patients
- The Roles and Responsibilities of a Consultant in Adult Psychiatry
- Safety for Trainees in Psychiatry
- The Second Report of the Royal College of Psychiatrists Special Committee on ECT
- Services for Younger People with Alzheimer's Disease and Other Dementias
- Sexual Abuse and Harassment in Psychiatric Settings

- Society and the Royal College of Psychiatrists
- Strategies for the Management of Disturbed and Violent Patients in Psychiatric Units
- Substance Misuse Detainees in Police Custody
- The Treatment of Perpetrators of Child Sexual Abuse
- Wish You Were Here? Ethical Considerations in the Admission of Patients to Substandard Psychiatric Units

Society for Academic Emergency Medicine
<http://www.saem.org>

Position Statements

- Emergency Medical Services Fellowship Guidelines
- Emergency Medicine Research Fellowship Guidelines
- Ethical Guidelines for Academic Emergency Physicians
- Response to Documentation Guidelines Modification
- Response to Practice Expense RVU Proposal
- Ultrasound Position Statement

Society for Adolescent Medicine
<http://www.adolescenthealth.org>

Position Papers

- Access to Health Care for Adolescents
- Adolescent Health Research Guidelines
- Clinical Preventive Services for Adolescents
- Code of Research Ethics
- Confidential Health Care for Adolescents
- Corporal Punishment in Schools
- Driver Education for Adolescents
- Eating Disorders in Adolescents
- Firearms and Adolescents
- HIV Infection and AIDS in Adolescents
- Homeless and Runaway Youth Health and Health Needs
- Incarcerated Youth
- Managed Care: Meeting the Health Care Needs of Adolescents
- Media and Contraception
- Reproductive Health Care for Adolescents
- School-Based Health Clinics
- Transition from Child-Centered to Adult Health Care Systems for Adolescents with Chronic Conditions

Position Statements

- Adolescent Inpatient Units
- Adolescent Medicine
- Hepatitis B Immunization
- Immunization of Adolescents
- Nutritional Health of Adolescents

Society for Developmental Biology
<http://sdbonline.org>

Position Statement

- Moratorium on Cloning of Human Beings

Society for General Microbiology
<http://www.socgenmicrobiol.org.uk>

Professional and Policy Matters

- Resistance to Antimicrobial Agents
- Safe Handling of Microorganisms and the Law

Society for Public Health Education
<http://www.sophe.org>

Resolutions

- To Promote a Comprehensive, Responsible National Tobacco Control Policy
- To Promote Public Health Through Physical Activity
- Provision of Health Education Programs Within Managed Care Organizations
- Resolution to Promote Fluoridation
- Role of Health Education in Preventing Firearm Injury

Society of American Gastrointestinal and Endoscopic Surgeons
<http://www.sages.org>

Position Statements

- Advanced Laparoscopic Training
- Concentration in General Surgery Residency
- Deep Venous Thrombosis Prophylaxis During Laparoscopic Surgery
- First Assistants
- Integrating Advanced Laparoscopy into Surgical Residency Training

- Laparoscopic Appendectomy
- New Procedures

Society of Critical Care Medicine
<http://www.sccm.org>

Position Statements
- Current Procedural Terminology
- Medicare Reform
- Reimbursement
- Universal Leukoreduction

Society of Diagnostic Medical Sonography
<http://www.sdms.org>

Position Statements
- Clinical Practice Standards
- Limited Exams
- National Minimum Standards for Diagnostic Ultrasound Professionals
- Nondiagnostic Use
- Scope of Practice
- Videotaping of OB Exams

Society of Emergency Medicine Physician Assistants
<http://www.sempa.org>

Issue Brief
- Physician Assistants and Emergency Medicine

Society of Gastroenterology Nurses and Associates
<http://www.sgna.org>

Position Statements
- Manipulation of Endoscopes During Endoscopic Procedures
- Performance of Flexible Sigmoidoscopy by Registered Nurses for the Purpose of Colorectal Screening
- Performance of Gastrointestinal Manometry Studies and Provocative Testing
- Placement of Percutaneous Endoscopic Gastrostomy (PEG) Tube
- Reuse of Single-Use Critical Medical Devices
- Role Delineation of Assistive Personnel

- Role Delineation of the Advanced-Practice Nurse in Gastroenterology/Hepatology and Endoscopy
- Role Delineation of the Licensed Practical/Vocational Nurse in Gastroenterology and/or Endoscopy
- Role Delineation of the Registered Nurse in a Staff Position in Gastroenterology and/or Endoscopy
- Safe Operation of Radiographic Equipment During GI Endoscopic Procedures
- Sedation and Analgesia

Society of General Internal Medicine
<http://www.sgim.org>

Issue Briefs

- Access to Care
- Health Services Research Funding
- Health Systems Reform
- Human Rights
- Managed Care
- Medicare/GME Funding
- SGIM Proposal for Medicare GME Reform
- Support the American Hospital Preservation Act
- Support the Medicaid Safety Net Hospital Preservation Act
- Primary Care
- Title VII (Health Professions Education)
- VA Medical Research

Society of Geriatric Cardiology
<http://www.sgcard.org>

Position Papers

- Physical Activity and Exercise Training in the Elderly
- Treatment of High Blood Pressure in the Elderly
- What Older Adults Should Know About High Cholesterol

Society of Interventional Radiology
<http://www.sirweb.org>

Position Statement

- Radiation Safety

Society of Invasive Cardiovascular Professionals
<http://www.sicp.com>

Position Statements
- Drug Testing of Health Care Professionals
- Entry of Health Professionals Who Practice in the Cardiac Catheterization Laboratory
- Ethics in Cardiology Research
- Hazards in the Cardiac Catheterization Lab
- Patient Advocacy
- Role Expectations for Cardiac Catheterization Lab Managers
- Staffing in the Cardiac Catheterization Lab

Society of Pediatric Nurses
<http://www.pedsnurses.org>

Position Statements/Action Plans
- Children, Violence, and Resiliency
- Immunizations
- Pediatric Firearm Injuries
- Pediatric Injury Prevention

Society of Thoracic Surgeons
<http://www.sts.org>

Position Papers
- The Role of Business Arrangements in the Care of Patients: A Review of Issues and the Ethics of the Hiring of Cardiothoracic Surgeons by Cardiology Practices
- STS Position on Negotiating Units for Physicians

Society of Toxicology
<http://www.toxicology.org>

Position Statements
- Animals in Research Public Policy Statement
- Guiding Principles in the Use of Animals in Toxicology
- Participation in Advisory Boards
- Principles for Research Priorities in Toxicology
- The Role of Government in Science Regulation
- The Safety of Genetically Modified Foods Produced Through Biotechnology
- Toxicologic Principles Do Not Support the Banning of Chlorine
- The Use of Animals in Toxicology

Vermont Medical Society
<http://www.vtmd.org>

Position Statement

- Physician-Assisted Suicide

Washington State Medical Association
<http://www.wsma.org>

Position Statements

- Abortion
- Abuse
- Access to Health Care (Health Care Reform)
- Accident Prevention
- Accreditation/Licensure
- Adolescent Care
- Aging
- AIDS/HIV
- Alcohol and Alcoholism
- Alternative Dispute Resolutions
- Artificial Insemination
- Benefits Packages
- Biomedical Research
- Birth Control
- Blood
- Cancer
- Capital Punishment
- Castration
- Chiropractors
- Clinical Investigation
- Clinical Laboratory Improvement Act
- Clinical Trials
- Confidentiality
- Contractual Relationships
- Corporal Punishment
- Data Collection
- Death/Dying
- Disciplinary Procedures
- Discipline and Medicine
- Discrimination
- Drugs—Regulation and Standardization
- Education

- Education—Medical
- Emergency Medical Services
- Environmental Health
- Fees
- Fetal Research
- Fireworks
- Foods and Nutrition
- Genetics
- Guns
- Health Care
- Health Manpower
- Home Health Care
- Hospitals
- Immunizations
- Impaired Physicians
- Informed Consent
- Insurance
- Labor and Industries Program
- Liability
- Liability Reform Positions
- Managed Care
- Maternal and Infant Health Care
- Medicaid
- Medical Boards
- Medical Directors
- Medical Ethics
- Medical Quality Assurance Commission
- Medicare
- Mental Health Care
- Migrant Workers
- Minority Health Care
- Nonscientific Practitioners
- Nursing
- Optometry
- Organs
- Patient
- Peer Review
- Physical Therapists
- Physician Advertising and Publicity
- Physician Assistants
- Physician Health Plan Participation
- Physician Practice

- Physician Profiling
- Physician Records
- Physician Rights and Responsibilities
- Physicians
- Political Action
- Prescribing Practices
- Prisons
- Professional Review Organization
- Public Health
- Research
- Retired Physicians
- Rural Health Care
- Scope of Practice
- Specialists
- Sports
- Surgery/Invasive Procedures
- Tax Reform
- Television
- Tobacco
- The Uninsured
- Veterans Medical Care
- Volunteerism
- War
- Washington State Bar Association
- Women's Health Care Issues
- Wrongful Birth/Wrongful Life

Washington State Public Health Association
<http://www.wspha.org>

Resolutions

- Access to Sterile Syringes and Needles
- Averting a Public Health Crisis Caused by Drug Shortages
- Breast Cancer Screening
- Calling Upon School Officials to Partner with Public Health Officials to Improve Student Children's Health Insurance Program
- Controlling Hepatitis A
- Diets, Dietary Messages, and Levels of Physical Activity
- Fluoridation of Public Water Systems
- Health Care 2000 Voter Initiative
- Hepatitis A Vaccination

- Life Jackets, Children, and Boats
- Opposing Initiative 695
- Preventing Human and Environmental Mercury Exposure and Harm
- Public Health Funding for a Safer, Healthier Washington
- Reduce the Incidence of Violence
- Reducing the Burden of Arthritis
- Resolution to Endorse Initiative 245
- Statewide Public Health Standards
- Support for Initiative 773—Tobacco Tax
- Tobacco Advertising
- Unintended Pregnancy
- Work-Related Musculoskeletal Disorders

West Virginia Hospital Association
<http://www.wvha.com>

Policy Statements

- Certificate of Need
- Children's Health Insurance Coverage
- Clean Indoor Air
- Credentialing
- Definition of Emergency
- Domestic Violence Education and Screening
- Elimination of Broad-Based Provider Taxes
- Elimination of Medicaid DSH Payments
- Expansion of Health Care
- Fair Payment Levels
- Health Care Liability Hospital Rate Setting
- Managed Care
- Medicaid Medical Errors
- Needles and "Sharps" Safety Devices
- PEIA Funding and Provider Payments
- Professional Licensing
- Representation versus Advocacy
- Tobacco Excise Tax Act
- Tobacco Settlement
- Unitary Drug Pricing
- Workforce Shortages and Staffing in Hospitals

Wisconsin Medical Society
<http://www.wisconsinmedicalsociety.org>

Policy Statements

- Abortion
- Accident/Injury Prevention
- AIDS
- Alcohol and Other Drug Abuse
- Alternative Medicine
- Antitrust Laws
- Cost Containment
- Data (Health Care)
- Data (Physician Specific)
- Drugs, Regulation and Standardization
- Education (Continuing Medical)
- Education (Medical)
- Education of Other Professionals
- Emergency Medicine
- Environmental/Occupational Health
- Ethics
- Extended Care Facilities
- Gambling
- Health System Reform
- Home Health
- Hospital Medical Staff
- Impaired Physicians
- Insurance: Coverage/Reimbursement/Mandates
- Interprofessional Relations
- Liability and Malpractice Issues
- Managed Care
- Maternal and Child Health
- Medical Care
- Medical Examining Board
- Medical Records
- Medicare and Medicaid
- Mental Health
- Nurses and Nursing
- Ophthalmology and Optometry
- Outreach (Medical)
- Partner Care
- Pharmacy
- Physically/Mentally Impaired

- Physician Extenders
- Physicians
- Practice Parameters
- Property Tax Exemptions
- Public Health/Safety
- Resource-Based Relative Value Scale (RBRVS)
- Review: Peer
- Review: Quality Assurance and Utilization
- Rural Health
- Safe Transportation
- School Health
- Scope of Practice
- Smoking and Tobacco
- Sports
- Tort Reform
- Underserved Areas
- Uninsured
- Violence

Wisconsin Public Health Association
<http://www.wpha.org>

Passed Resolutions/Position Papers

- Access to Therapeutic Marijuana/Cannabis
- Database on Pesticide Use in Wisconsin
- Dedication of Tobacco Settlement Dollars to Tobacco Control and Prevention Initiatives
- Development of Successful Comprehensive Home Visitation Programs
- Environmental Health
- Government Insurance Programs in Wisconsin
- Insurance Coverage for Immunization of Children
- International Injury and Violence
- Legislation to Lower Blood Alcohol Content Illegal for Motor Vehicle Drivers
- Oppose Budget Provision That Bypasses Voters and Public Service Commission in the Sale of Utilities
- Preventing Youth Violence in Wisconsin
- Prevention of Intentional Injuries and Violence
- Prevention of Lead Poisoning
- Principles of State or National Health Care Programs
- Promote Passage of the Public Health Statutes

- Public Health Information System in Wisconsin
- Public Officials in the Conduct of Their Work Duties
- Resolution Calling for a Separate Department of Health
- Resolution Calling for Base Funding for Core Public Health Services Under Health Care Reform
- Resolution in Support of Intent of 1997 AB 2000 to Reinstate the Exemption from Trespass Laws
- Resolution in Support of Raising the Cigarette Tax
- Resolution in Support of Right from the Start Initiative
- Resolution Mandating the Use of Helmets by All Bicyclists
- Resolution on Preadolescent Hep B Vaccination
- Resolution Promoting Passage of AB 167 (Licensure of Dietitians)
- Resolution Recognizing Campaign Finance Reform As a Public Health Priority
- Resolution Regarding Mouth Guard Use for Prevention of Orofacial Injuries
- Resolution Supporting Maintaining the Age of 21 As the Mandatory Drinking Age
- Resolution to Prevent Tobacco Industry Influence in WPHA
- Resolution to Support Funding for Core Public Health Services
- Resolution to Support Harm Reduction Programs to Reduce the Transmission of HIV and Other Disease
- Resolution to Support Improvements in Dental Care Access
- Resolution to Support the Office of the Surgeon General
- Revision of Wisconsin's Public Health Statutes
- Support a State Policy That Will Assure the Scheduled and Timely Release of Vital Records
- Support Clean Indoor Air Through Elimination of Environmental Tobacco Smoke
- Support for Regulation of Media Programming
- Support of Healthier People in Wisconsin: A Public Health Agenda for the Year 2000
- In Support of Technical and Professional Staffing in the Wisconsin Division of Health
- Support Statewide Ban on Sale of Home-Use Mercury Thermometers
- Use of Latex Products in Settings Where Health Care Is Provided
- Wisconsin Arthritis Action Plan

World Medical Association
<http://www.wma.net/e>

Position Statements

- Abuse
- Academic
- Access
- Accountability
- Addicts
- Adolescent
- Advertising
- Advocacy
- Afghanistan
- AIDS
- Alcohol
- Animal
- Antimicrobial Drug
- Armed Conflict
- Autonomy
- Biological Weapons
- Biomedical Research
- Body Search
- Boxing
- Boycott
- Care
- Chemical
- Child
- Child Abuse
- Chronic
- Cloning
- Code
- Computers
- Condemnation
- Confidentiality
- Conflict
- Contraception
- Control
- Counselling
- Crime
- Cruel
- Databases
- Death

- Degrading
- Demographic
- Detention
- Disasters
- Drug
- Elderly
- Embargoes
- Embryo
- Engineering
- Environment
- Ethics
- Euthanasia
- Export Tobacco
- Family
- Female
- Fertilization
- Fetal Tissue
- Flights
- Freedom
- Generic Drug
- Genctic
- Geneva
- Genital
- Genome
- Group Practice
- Hague
- Hamburg
- Hazard
- Health
- Health Care
- Health Hazard
- Health Professionals
- Health Promotion
- Helsinki
- HIV
- Home Medical Monitoring
- Hong Kong
- Human Genome
- Human Organ Transplantation
- Human Rights
- Hunger
- Import Tobacco

- Imprisonment
- Improvement in Health Care
- Independence
- Infant
- Inhuman
- Injections
- Injury
- Integrity
- International
- Investment
- In Vitro
- Karadzic
- Kosovo
- Land Mines
- Licensing
- Life
- Lisbon
- Live Organ
- Malpractice
- Malta
- Manpower
- Manufacture of Tobacco
- Medical Care
- Medical Doctors
- Medical Education
- Medical Ethics
- Medical Group Practice
- Medical Malpractice
- Medical Manpower
- Medical Meetings
- Medical Monitoring
- Medical Practitioners
- Medical Process
- Medical Schools
- Medical Technology
- Medical Therapy
- Mental Illness
- Mines
- Mutilation
- Neglect
- Noise Pollution
- Nuclear Weapons

- Opiate Drugs
- Organ Trade
- Organ Transplantation
- Oslo
- Ottawa
- Outpatient Treatment
- Pain
- Patents
- Patient
- Peace
- Persistent Vegetative State
- Pharmacists
- Physician
- Planning
- Political
- Pollution
- Practice
- Prescription
- Prison
- Prisoners
- Professional
- Promotion
- Prosecution
- Provision
- Psychotropic Drugs
- Punishment
- Quality
- Radovan Karadzic
- Rancho Mirage
- Rapporteur
- Reduction
- Refugees
- Regulations
- Research
- Resistance
- Responsibility
- Rights
- Road Safety

- Role of Physicians
- Rural Areas
- Safety
- Sale of Tobacco
- Sanction
- Search
- Self-Medication
- Self-Regulation
- SIrUS Project
- Smoking
- Sports Medicine
- Standards
- Strike
- Substitution
- Suicide
- Sydney
- Telemedicine
- Terminal Illness
- Testing
- Therapeutic
- Time of Armed Conflict
- Tobacco
- Tokyo
- Torture
- Trade
- Traffic Injury
- Transplantation
- Treatment
- Tuberculosis
- United Nations
- Vegetative State
- Venice
- Violation
- Violence
- War
- Weapons
- Women
- Workforce
- Workplace

Wound, Ostomy and Continence Nurses Society
<http://www.wocn.org>

Position Statements

- Conservative Sharp Wound Debridement for Registered Nurses
- Coverage for Pelvic Floor Biofeedback Therapy
- Role of Wound, Ostomy, and Continence Nurses in Continence Management
- Staging Pressure Ulcers

Appendix A

Biomedical Organizations Without Position Documents

Aboriginal Nurses Association of Canada
Academic Orthopaedic Society
Academy for Eating Disorders
Academy for Implants and Transplants
Academy for the Study of the Psychoanalytic Arts
Academy of Ambulatory Foot and Ankle Surgery
Academy of Behavioral Medicine Research
Academy of Clinical Psychology
Academy of Counseling Psychology
Academy of Dental Materials
Academy of Dental Sleep Medicine
Academy of Dentistry for Persons with Disabilities
Academy of Dentistry International
Academy of Dispensing Audiologists
Academy of Forensic and Industrial Chiropractic Consultants
Academy of General Dentistry
Academy of Laser Dentistry
Academy of Operative Dentistry
Academy of Oral Dynamics
Academy of Organizational and Occupational Psychiatry
Academy of Osseointegration
Academy of Psychological Clinical Science
Academy of Radiology Research
Academy of Rehabilitative Audiology

Note: As of the date of publication, these organizations were found not to have position documents, either because they were not found on their Web sites, because an official e-mail from the organization indicated that, or because the organization does not have a Web presence. However, readers are encouraged to visit organization Web sites as in the future such documents may be posted for public review. In addition, many organizations revise or establish new Web sites and post documents heretofore not available.

Academy of Surgical Research
Academy of Upper Cervical Chiropractic Organizations
Acoustic Neuroma Association
Acupuncture and Oriental Medicine Alliance
Acupuncture Medical Association of Thailand
Aerospace Medical Association of Korea
African Association of Dermatology
African Association of Nephrology
African Gerontological Society
Age Anesthesia Association
Alabama Academy of Family Physicians
Alabama Academy of General Dentistry
Alaska Dental Society
Alaska Public Health Association
Alberta Medical Review Officers
Allergy Society of South Africa
Alliance for the Prudent Use of Antibiotics
Alliance of Cardiovascular Professionals
All India Ophthalmological Association
Alps Adria Society for Immunology of Reproduction
Alternative Health Professionals Association
Alternative Medicine Foundation
Ambulatory Pediatric Association
American Academy for Cerebral Palsy and Developmental Medicine
American Academy of Allergy and Asthma and Immunology
American Academy of Alternative Medicine
American Academy of Ambulatory Care
American Academy of Ambulatory Care Nursing
American Academy of Ambulatory Foot Surgery
American Academy of Anesthesiologists Assistants
American Academy of Cardiovascular Perfusion
American Academy of Clinical Neuropsychology
American Academy of Clinical Psychiatrists
American Academy of Clinical Toxicology
American Academy of Cosmetic Dentistry
American Academy of Cosmetic Surgery
American Academy of Craniofacial Pain
American Academy of Dental Practice Administration
American Academy of Dermatology
American Academy of Environmental Medicine
American Academy of Esthetic Dentistry
American Academy of Experts in Traumatic Stress

American Academy of Facial Plastic and Reconstructive Surgery
American Academy of Fixed Prosthodontics
American Academy of Forensic Psychology
American Academy of Gnathologic Orthopedics
American Academy of Health Behavior
American Academy of Health Care Providers—Addictive Disorders
American Academy of Health Physics
American Academy of Home Care Physicians
American Academy of Implant Dentistry
American Academy of Industrial Hygiene
American Academy of Maxillofacial Prosthetics
American Academy of Neurological and Orthopaedic Surgeons
American Academy of Neurological Surgery
American Academy of Neurology
American Academy of Orthodontics for the General Dentist
American Academy of Orthopedic Manual Physical Therapy
American Academy of Osteopathy
American Academy of Otolaryngology—Head and Neck Surgery
American Academy of Pain Management
American Academy of Pharmaceutical Physicians
American Academy of Physical Therapy
American Academy of Podiatric Practice Management
American Academy of Podiatric Sports Medicine
American Academy of Private Practice in Speech Pathology and Audiology
American Academy of Psychoanalysis
American Academy of Psychotherapists
American Academy of Restorative Dentistry
American Academy of Sanitarians
American Academy of Somnology
American Academy of Tropical Medicine
American Academy of Wound Management
American Acupuncture Association
American Aging Association
American Allergy Association
American Alternative Medicine Association
American Apitherapy Association
American Association for Aerosol Research
American Association for Applied and Therapeutic Humor
American Association for Cancer Research
American Association for Chronic Fatigue Syndrome
American Association for Clinical Chemistry
American Association for Emergency Psychiatry

American Association for Functional Orthodontics
American Association for Hand Surgery
American Association for Psychology and the Performing Arts
American Association for Respiratory Care
American Association for Technology in Psychiatry
American Association for the Study of Liver Diseases
American Association for the Surgery of Trauma
American Association for Thoracic Surgery
American Association for Women Podiatrists
American Association for Women Radiologists
American Association for World Health
American Association of Academic Chief Residents in Radiology
American Association of Anatomists
American Association of Blood Banks
American Association of Certified Allergists
American Association of Certified Orthoptists
American Association of Clinical Anatomists
American Association of Clinical Urologists
American Association of Colleges of Pharmacy
American Association of Colleges of Podiatric Medicine
American Association of Drugless Practitioners
American Association of Endocrine Surgeons
American Association of Eye and Ear Hospitals
American Association of Genito-Urinary Surgeons
American Association of Gynecologic Laparoscopists
American Association of Hip and Knee Surgeons
American Association of Hospital and Healthcare Podiatrists
American Association of Hospital Dentists
American Association of Hospital Podiatrists
American Association of Immunologists
American Association of Integrative Medicine
American Association of Internal Medicine
American Association of Kidney Patients
American Association of Managed Care Nurses
American Association of Medical Assistants
American Association of Medical Review Officers
American Association of Naturopathic Physicians
American Association of Neuropathologists
American Association of Neuroscience Nurses
American Association of Nurse Anesthetists
American Association of Nutritional Consultants
American Association of Office Nurses

American Association of Oriental Medicine
American Association of Orthodontists
American Association of Orthopaedic Foot and Ankle Surgeons
American Association of Orthopaedic Medicine
American Association of Pharmaceutical Scientists
American Association of Pharmacy Technicians
American Association of Physicists in Medicine
American Association of Poison Control Centers
American Association of Professional Hypnotherapists
American Association of Professional Ringside Physicians
American Association of Psychiatric Technicians
American Association of Public Health Physicians
American Association of Women Dentists
American Association of Women Podiatrists
American Autoimmune Related Diseases Association
American Biological Safety Association
American Black Chiropractic Association
American Board for Occupational Health Nurses
American Board of Abdominal Surgery
American Board of Allergy and Immunology
American Board of Alternative Medicine
American Board of Anesthesiology
American Board of Cardiovascular Perfusion
American Board of Chelation Therapy
American Board of Colon and Rectal Surgery
American Board of Dental Public Health
American Board of Dermatology
American Board of Emergency Medicine
American Board of Endodontics
American Board of Environmental Medicine
American Board of Facial Plastic and Reconstructive Surgery
American Board of Family Practice
American Board of Forensic Pathology
American Board of Genetic Counseling
American Board of Health Physics
American Board of Independent Medical Examiners
American Board of Industrial Hygiene
American Board of Managed Care Nursing
American Board of Medical Genetics
American Board of Medical Specialties
American Board of Neurological Surgery
American Board of Neuroscience Nursing

American Board of Nuclear Medicine
American Board of Nursing Specialties
American Board of Nutrition
American Board of Obstetrics and Gynecology
American Board of Ophthalmology
American Board of Opticianry
American Board of Orthopaedic Surgery
American Board of Otolaryngology
American Board of Pain Medicine
American Board of Pathology
American Board of Pediatrics
American Board of Physical Medicine and Rehabilitation
American Board of Plastic Surgery
American Board of Podiatric Surgery
American Board of Preventive Medicine
American Board of Professional Neuropsychology
American Board of Professional Psychology
American Board of Psychiatry and Neurology
American Board of Radiology
American Board of Sleep Medicine
American Board of Thoracic Surgery
American Board of Toxicology
American Board of Urology
American Chiropractic Association
American Chiropractic College of Radiology
American Chiropractic Rehabilitation Board
American Clinical Neurophysiology Society
American College for Advancement in Medicine
American College of Acupuncture and Oriental Medicine
American College of Chest Physicians
American College of Clinical Pharmacology
American College of Dentists
American College of Eye Surgeons
American College of Foot and Ankle Orthopedics and Medicine
American College of Foot and Ankle Pediatrics
American College of Foot and Ankle Surgeons
American College of Gastroenterology
American College of International Physicians
American College of Legal Medicine
American College of Mohs Micrographic Surgery and Cutaneous Oncology
American College of Neuropsychopharmacology

American College of Nuclear Medicine
American College of Nuclear Physicians
American College of Nutrition
American College of Obstetricians and Gynecologists
American College of Osteopathic Pediatricians
American College of Phlebology
American College of Physician Executives
American College of Podiatric Medical Review
American College of Prehospital Medicine
American College of Prosthodontists
American College of Radiation Oncology
American Conference of Governmental Industrial Hygienists
American Congress on Rehabilitation Medicine
American Council of the Blind
American Council on Pharmaceutical Education
American Council on Science and Health
American Dance Therapy Association
American Dental Assistants Association
American Dental Society of Anesthesiology
American Dental Trade Association
American Dietetic Association
American Endodontic Society
American Evaluation Association
American Foundation for AIDS Research
American Fracture Association
American Group Psychotherapy Association
American Headache Society
American Head and Neck Society
American Healthcare Radiology Administrators
American Health Information Management Association
American Health Quality Association
American Hepato-Pancreato-Billiary Association
American Holistic Health Association
American Holistic Medical Association
American Holistic Nurses Association
American Hyperlexia Association
American Independent Dentists Association
American Infertility Association
American Institute of Homeopathy
American Integrative Medical Association
American International Health Alliance
American International Health Council

American Laryngological Association
American Long-Term and Sub Acute Nurses Association
American Massage Therapy Association
American Mental Health Counselors Association
American Music Therapy Association
American Neurological Association
American Neuropsychiatric Association
American Occupational Therapy Association
American Optometric Association
American Orthopaedic Association
American Orthopaedic Society for Sports Medicine
American Orthopedic Rugby Football Association
American Orthoptic Council
American Osteopathic Association
American Osteopathic College of Dermatology
American Osteopathic College of Ophthalmology
American Osteopathic College of Otolaryngology—Head and Neck Surgery
American Osteopathic College of Radiology
American Otological Society
American Pediatric Society/Society for Pediatric Research
American Pediatric Surgery Association
American Pediatric Surgical Nurses Association
American Physiological Society
American Podiatric Medical Association
American Podiatric Medical Specialties Board
American Podiatric Medical Students Association
American Preventive Medical Association
American Psychoanalytic Association
American Psychological Association
American Psychological Society
American Psychotherapy and Medical Hypnosis Association
American Radiological Nurses Association
American Rhinologic Society
American Roentgen Ray Society
American School Food Service Association
American Sickle Cell Anemia Association
American Society for Aesthetic Plastic Surgery
American Society for Artificial Internal Organs
American Society for Automation in Pharmacy
American Society for Bariatric Surgery
American Society for Bone and Mineral Research

American Society for Clinical Investigation
American Society for Clinical Pharmacology and Therapeutics
American Society for Dental Aesthetics
American Society for Geriatric Dentistry
American Society for Healthcare Engineering
American Society for Healthcare Risk Management
American Society for Histocompatability and Immunogenics
American Society for Laser Medicine and Surgery
American Society for Neurochemistry
American Society for Psychosocial and Behavioral Oncology
American Society for Surgery of the Hand
American Society for Therapeutic Radiology and Oncology
American Society for Virology
American Society of Aerospace Medicine Specialists
American Society of Alternative Therapists
American Society of Anesthesia Technologists and Technicians
American Society of Anesthesiologists
American Society of Biomechanics
American Society of Clinical Hypnosis
American Society of Clinical Pathologists
American Society of Contemporary Medicine, Surgery, and Ophthalmology
American Society of Critical Care Anesthesiologists
American Society of Dentist Anesthesiologists
American Society of Dentistry for Children
American Society of Echocardiography
American Society of Emergency Radiology
American Society of Extra-Corporeal Technology
American Society of Forensic Odontology
American Society of Gastrointestinal Endoscopy
American Society of Head and Neck Radiology
American Society of Hypertension
American Society of Master Dental Technologists
American Society of Nephrology
American Society of Neurophysiological Monitoring
American Society of Neuroradiology
American Society of Ophthalmic Plastic and Reconstructive Surgery
American Society of Ophthalmic Registered Nurses
American Society of Orthopedic Professionals
American Society of Parasitologists
American Society of Pediatric Hematology/Oncology
American Society of Pediatric Nephrology

American Society of Pediatric Neuroradiology
American Society of Pediatric Otolaryngology
American Society of Pharmacognosy
American Society of Plastic Surgical Nurses
American Society of Podiatric Dermatology
American Society of Podiatric Medical Assistants
American Society of Psychoanalytic Physicians
American Society of Regional Anesthesia and Pain Medicine
American Society of Spine Radiology
American Society of Transplantation
American Society of Transplant Surgeons
American Society of Tropical Medicine and Hygiene
American Spinal Injury Association
American Sports Medicine Institute
American Thoracic Society
American Tinnitus Association
American Trauma Society
Anaerobe Society of the Americas
Anatomical Society of Great Britain and Ireland
Anesthesiologists Independent Practitioners Association
Anesthetic Research Society
Angiogenesis Foundation
Anxiety Disorders Association of America
Applied Psychometrics Society
Arizona Academy of Family Physicians
Arizona Hospital and Healthcare Association
Arizona Medical Association
Arizona Osteopathic Medical Association
Arizona Public Health Association
Arizona Society of Echocardiography
Arkansas Academy of Family Physicians
Arkansas Hospital Association
Arkansas Medical Society
Armed Forces Infectious Diseases Society
Arthroscopy Association of North America
Asia and Oceania Thyroid Association
Asian American Psychological Association
Asian Association for Dynamic Osteosynthesis
Asian Dermatological Association
Asian Pacific Endodontic Confederation
Asian Pacific Society for Neurochemistry
Asian Sleep Research Society

Asian Society for Cardiovascular Surgery
Asian Society for Emergency Medicine
Asian Society for Female Urology
Asian Surgical Association
Asia Pacific Orthopaedic Association
Association for Academic Psychiatry
Association for Advanced Training in the Behavioral Sciences
Association for Advancement of Behavior Therapy
Association for Applied Psychophysiology and Biofeedback
Association for Australian Rural Nurses
Association for Behavior Analysis
Association for Child Psychoanalysis
Association for Comprehensive Neurotherapy
Association for European Pediatric Cardiologists
Association for Hospital Medical Education
Association for Humanistic Psychology
Association for Integrative Medicine
Association for Low Flow Anesthesia
Association for Macular Diseases
Association for Medical Education and Research in Substance Abuse
Association for Psychological Type
Association for Research in Nervous and Mental Disease
Association for Research in Otolaryngology
Association for Specialists in Group Work
Association for the Advancement of Applied Sport Psychology
Association for the Advancement of Gestalt Therapy
Association for the Advancement of Philosophy and Psychiatry
Association for the Advancement of Psychology
Association for the Scientific Study of Consciousness
Association for the Study and Application of the Methods of Ilizarov
Association for Traumatic Stress Specialists
Association for Treatment and Training in the Attachment of Children
Association of Anesthesia Clinical Directors
Association of Anesthetists of Great Britain and Ireland
Association of Aviation Medical Examiners
Association of Behavioral Healthcare Executives
Association of Black Cardiologists
Association of Black Psychologists
Association of Bone and Joint Surgeons
Association of British Neurologists
Association of Cardiothoracic Anaesthetists
Association of Child Neurology Nurses

Association of Children's Prosthetic-Orthotic Clinics
Association of Clinical Cytogeneticists
Association of Clinical Research Professionals
Association of Clinicians for the Underserved
Association of European Pediatric Cardiology
Association of Family Practice Administrators
Association of Family Practice Residency Directors
Association of Genetic Nurses and Counselors
Association of Genetic Technologists
Association of Managed Care Dentists
Association of Medical Microbiologists
Association of Medicine and Psychiatry
Association of Military Osteopathic Physicians and Surgeons
Association of Military Surgeons of the United States
Association of National Health Service Occupational Physicians
Association of Natural Medicine Pharmacists
Association of Neurosurgical Physician Assistants
Association of Obstetrics and Gynecology of the Republic of China
Association of Occupational and Environmental Clinics
Association of Occupational Therapists in Mental Health
Association of Ottawa Anesthesiologists
Association of Paediatric Anaesthetists of Great Britain and Ireland
Association of Palliative Medicine
Association of Pediatric Oncology Nurses
Association of Physician Assistants in Cardiovascular Surgery
Association of Police Surgeons
Association of Polysomnographic Technologists
Association of Preventive Medicine Residents
Association of Professors of Gynecology and Obstetrics
Association of Professors of Medicine
Association of Program Directors in Internal Medicine
Association of Renal Technicians UK
Association of Residents in Radiation Oncology
Association of Resuscitation Training Officers
Association of Societies for Occupational Safety and Health
Association of State and Territorial Dental Directors
Association of Surgeons in Training
Association of Surgeons of Great Britain and Ireland
Association of Teachers of Preventive Medicine
Association of Traditional Health Practitioners
Association of University Radiologists
Association of Vascular and Interventional Radiographers

Association of Volleyball Medical Doctors
Association of Women Surgeons
Australasian Association of Paediatric Surgeons
Australasian Faculty of Occupational Medicine
Australasian Sleep Association
Australasian Society for Cardio-Vascular Perfusionists
Australasian Society for Emergency Medicine
Australasian Society for Immunology
Australasian Society for Infectious Disease
Australasian Society of Blood Transfusion
Australasian Society of Cardiac and Thoracic Surgeons
Australasian Society of Human Genetics
Australian Acupuncture and Chinese Medicine Association
Australian and New Zealand Intensive Care Society
Australian and New Zealand Society for Cell and Developmental Biology
Australian and New Zealand Society of Occupational Medicine
Australian Association for Exercise and Sports Science
Australian Association of Neurologists
Australian Atherosclerosis Society
Australian College of Critical Care Nurses
Australian College of Dermatologists
Australian College of Occupational Health Nurses
Australian College of Rural and Remote Medicine
Australian Dental Association
Australian Healthcare Association
Australian Hospital Association
Australian Infection Control Association
Australian Neuroscience Society
Australian Orthopaedic Association
Australian Physiotherapy Association
Australian Society for Biochemistry and Molecular Biology
Australian Society for Microbiology
Australian Society of Forensic Dentistry
Australian Society of Gynaecologic Oncologists
Australian Society of Orthodontists
Australian Traditional Medicine Society
Austrian Society for Aerospace Medicine
Austrian Society for Allergology and Immunology
Austrian Society for Human Genetics
Austrian Society of Neurosurgery
Aviation Medical Society of Australia and New Zealand
Baromedical Nurses Association

Behavioral Toxicology Society
Behavior Genetics Association
Belgian Arthroscopy Association
Belgian Association for Cardio-Thoracic Surgery
Belgian Association for Urological Nurses and Associates
Belgian Association of Pediatric Orthopaedics
Belgian Society of Biochemistry and Molecular Biology
Belgian Society of Cardiology
Belgian Society of Neurosurgery
Belgian Society of Periodontology
Belgium Hospital Association
Biophysical Society
Brain Tumor Society
Brazilian Intensive Care Society
Brazilian Medical Society
Brazilian Society for Cardiovascular Surgery
Brazilian Society for Lower Genital Tract Pathology and Colposcopy
Brazilian Society of Nephrology
Brazilian Society of Plastic Surgery
Breast Cancer Society of Canada
British and Irish Pain Society
British Andrology Association
British Association for Accident and Emergency Medicine
British Association for Cardiac Rehabilitation
British Association for Immediate Care
British Association for Pediatric Otolaryngology
British Association for Surgery of the Knee
British Association for the Study of Community Dentistry
British Association of Aesthetic Plastic Surgeons
British Association of Audiological Physicians
British Association of Clinical Anatomists
British Association of Dermatologists
British Association of Occupational Therapists
British Association of Oral Maxillofacial Surgeons
British Association of Plastic Surgeons
British Association of Sport and Exercise Sciences
British Association of Urological Surgeons
British Biophysical Society
British Blood Transfusion Society
British Cardiac Society
British Chiropractic Association
British Columbia Physiotherapy Association

British Endodontic Society
British Epilepsy Association
British Heart Foundation
British Herbal Medicine Association
British Homeopathic Association
British Institute of Radiology
British Medical Association—Northern Ireland
British Medical Association—Scotland
British Medical Association—Wales
British Medical Laser Association
British Medical Ultrasound Society
British Menopause Society
British Neuroendocrine Group
British Neuropathological Society
British Neuroscience Association
British Nuclear Medicine Society
British Occupational Hygiene Society
British Ophthalmic Anesthesia Society
British Orthodontic Society
British Orthopaedic Foot Surgery Society
British Orthopaedic Sports Trauma Association
British Orthopaedic Trainees Association
British Paediatric Immunology and Infectious Diseases Group
British Pharmacological Society
British Psychological Society
British Society for Allergy and Clinical Immunology
British Society for Antimicrobial Chemotherapy
British Society for Cell Biology
British Society for Children's Orthopaedic Surgery
British Society for Dental Research
British Society for Developmental Biology
British Society for Disability and Oral Health
British Society for Haematology
British Society for Histocompatability and Immunogenetics
British Society for Immunology
British Society for Parasitology
British Society for Restorative Dentistry
British Society for Rheumatology
British Society for Surgery of the Hand
British Society of Audiology
British Society of Gastroenterology
British Society of Medical and Dental Hypnosis

British Society of Orthopaedic Anaesthetists
British Society of Pediatric Endocrinology
British Society of Periodontology
British Thyroid Foundation
Bulgarian Society for Immunology of Reproduction
California Academy of Ophthalmology
California Association of Neurological Surgeons
California Association of Nurse Anesthetists
California Association of Orthodontists
California Dental Association
California Healthcare Association
California Medical Association
California Pediatric Society
California Pharmacists Association
California Physical Therapy Association
California Primary Care Association
California Radiological Society
California Society for Cardiac Rehabilitation
California Society of Anesthesiologists
California Society of Pediatric Dentists
California Society of Periodontists
California Society of Plastic Surgeons
California State Association of Occupational Health Nurses
California Urological Association
Calorie Control Council
Canadian Academy of Endodontics
Canadian Academy of Geriatric Psychiatry
Canadian Academy of Manipulative Therapy
Canadian Academy of Periodontology
Canadian Academy of Psychiatry and Law
Canadian Academy of Restorative Dentistry and Prosthodontics
Canadian Academy of Sport Medicine
Canadian Association for Anatomy, Neurobiology and Cell Biology
Canadian Association for Clinical Microbiology and Infectious Diseases
Canadian Association for Health, Physical Education, Recreation and Dance
Canadian Association for the Study of the Liver
Canadian Association of Cardiac Rehabilitation
Canadian Association of Emergency Physicians
Canadian Association of Gastroenterology
Canadian Association of Medical Oncologists
Canadian Association of Medical Radiation Technologists

Canadian Association of Neuropathologists
Canadian Association of Nurses in Oncology
Canadian Association of Optometrists
Canadian Association of Oral and Maxillofacial Surgeons
Canadian Association of Orthodontists
Canadian Association of Pathologists
Canadian Association of Pharmacy in Oncology
Canadian Association of Physical Medicine and Rehabilitation
Canadian Association of Radiologists
Canadian Collaborative Group for Cancer Genetics
Canadian College of Physicists in Medicine
Canadian Critical Care Society
Canadian Dental Association
Canadian Fertility and Andrology Society
Canadian Interventional Radiology Association
Canadian Laser Aesthetic Surgery Society
Canadian Melanoma Foundation
Canadian Mental Health Association
Canadian Physiotherapy Association
Canadian Psychological Association
Canadian Sleep Society
Canadian Society for Biomechanics
Canadian Society for Brain, Behaviour and Cognitive Science
Canadian Society for Clinical Investigation
Canadian Society for Epidemiology and Biostatistics
Canadian Society for Vascular Surgeons
Canadian Society for Vascular Surgery
Canadian Society of Atherosclerosis, Thrombosis and Vascular Biology
Canadian Society of Clinical Perfusion
Canadian Society of Diagnostic Medical Sonographers
Canadian Society of Immunology
Canadian Society of Internal Medicine
Canadian Society of Microbiologists
Canadian Society of Nephrology
Canadian Society of Otolaryngologists
Canadian Society of Plastic Surgeons
Canadian Society of Respiratory Therapists
Canadian Society of Surgical Oncology
Canadian Thoracic Society
Canadian Thyroid Association
Cancer Control Society
Cardiac Society of Australia and New Zealand

Cardiovascular and Interventional Radiological Society of Europe
Case Management Society of America
Catholic Health Association
Cell Death Society
Central Australian Rural Practitioners Association
Central States Occupational Medical Association
Chartered Society of Physiotherapy
Child Neurology Society
Children's Craniofacial Association
Chilean Society of Nephrology
China International Travel Healthcare Association
Chinese Epidemiological Association
Chinese Medical Association
Chinese Society for Microbiology
Chinese Taipei Association of Family Medicine
Chiropractic Association of Ireland
Christian Dental Association
Civil Aviation Medical Association
Clerkship Directors in Internal Medicine
Clinical Genetics Society
Clinical Immunology Society
Clinical Laboratory Management Association
Clinical Ligand Assay Society
Clinical Magnetic Resonance Society
Clinical Molecular Genetics Society
Cognitive Neuroscience Society
College of American Pathology
College of Family Physicians of Singapore
College of Healthcare Information Management Executives
College of Optometrists in Vision Development
Colombian Association of Neurosurgery
Colorado Academy of Family Physicians
Colorado Association of Nurse Anesthetists
Colorado Dental Association
Colorado Orthopaedic Society
Colorado Public Health Association
Commonwealth Dental Association
Community and Hospital Infection Control Association of Canada
Complementary Medical Association
Confederation of German Anesthesiologists
Connecticut Association for Healthcare Quality
Connecticut College of Emergency Physicians

Connecticut Hospital Association
Connecticut Primary Care Association
Connecticut Society of Perfusion
Connecticut State Dental Association
Connecticut State Medical Society
Connecticut State Society of Anesthesiologists
Conservative Orthopedics International Association
Controlled Release Society
Council for International Organizations of Medical Sciences
Council for Responsible Nutrition
Council of Medical Genetics Organizations
Council of Medical Specialty Societies
Council on Chiropractic Orthopedics
Creutzfeldt-Jakob Disease Foundation
Croatian Neurosurgical Society
Czech Association of Anesthesia, Resuscitation, and Intensive Medicine
Czech Gynecological and Obstetrical Society
Czech Society of Cardiology
Czech Society of Medical Genetics
Czech Urological Society
Danish Endocrine Society
Danish Epidemiological Society
Danish Incontinence Association
Danish Medical Association
Danish Neurosurgical Society
Danish Society for Extracorporeal Circulation
Danish Society for Immunology
Danish Society for Vascular Surgery
Danish Society of Hematology
Danish Society of Nephrology
Danish Society of Radiology
Danish Urological Society
Delaware Healthcare Association
Delaware Medical Society
Delaware Occupational Therapy Association
Delaware Public Health Association
Delaware Society for Respiratory Care
Delhi Opthalmological Society
Dental Anthropology Association
Dermatological Society of Thailand
Difficult Airway Society
District of Columbia Dental Society

District of Columbia Medical Society
Doctors Against Handgun Injury
Drug Information Association
Dutch Association of Environmental Medicine
Dutch Association of Pediatric Anaesthetists
Dutch Society for Sleep-Wake Research
Eastern Association for the Surgery of Trauma
Eastern Dental Society
Eastern Psychological Association
Eastern Society for Pediatric Research
Egyptian Dental Association
Egyptian Hypertension Society
Egyptian Orthodontic Society
Egyptian Orthopedic Association
Egyptian Periodontal Restorative Society
Egyptian Society for Joint Diseases and Arthritis
Egyptian Society of Plastic and Reconstructive Surgeons
Endocrine Society
Endometriosis Association
Endourological Society
Endourology Society
Environmental Illness Society of Canada
Environmental Mutagen Society
European Academy of Allergology and Clinical Immunology
European Academy of Anesthesiology
European Academy of Dermatology
European Academy of Esthetic Dentistry
European Academy of Otology and Neuro-otology
European Alliance of Neuromuscular Disorder Associations
European Association for Cancer Research
European Association for Cardio-thoracic Surgery
European Association for Dental Public Health
European Association for Endoscopic Surgery
European Association for Osseointegration
European Association for the Study of Diabetes
European Association for the Treatment of Addiction
European Association for Vision and Eye Research
European Association of Cardiothoracic Anesthesiologists
European Association of Neurosurgical Societies
European Association of Personality Psychology
European Association of Plastic Surgeons
European Association of Psychological Assessment

European Association of Urology
European Association of Vascular Surgeons in Training
European Atherosclerosis Society
European Brief Therapy Association
European Calcified Tissue Society
European College of Sport Science
European Confederation of Neuropathological Societies
European Congress of Radiology
European Council for Classical Homeopathy
European Federation for Experimental Morphology
European Federation of Endocrinology Societies
European Federation of Periodontology
European Health Psychology Society
European Oncology Nursing Society
European Ophthalmic Pathology Society
European Paediatric Orthopaedic Society
European Renal Association—European Dialysis and Transplant Association
European Rural and Isolated Practitioners Association
European Sleep Research Society
European Society for Clinical Virology
European Society for Dermatological Research
European Society for Emergency Medicine
European Society for Human Reproduction and Embryology
European Society for Immunodeficiencies
European Society for Intravenous Anesthesia
European Society for Magnetic Resonance in Medicine and Biology
European Society for Neurochemistry
European Society for Neurogastroenterology and Motility
European Society for Noninvasive Cardiovascular Dynamics
European Society for Paediatric Infectious Disease
European Society for Pediatric Endocrinology
European Society for Pediatric Nephrology/European Society for Pediatric Urology
European Society for Primary Care Gastroenterology
European Society for Sexual and Impotence Research
European Society for Therapeutic Radiology and Oncology
European Society of Anaesthesiologists
European Society of Biochemical Pharmacology
European Society of Biomechanics
European Society of Breast Imaging
European Society of Cataract and Refractive Surgery

European Society of Clinical Microbiology and Infectious Diseases
European Society of Clinical Pharmacy
European Society of Contraception
European Society of Gastrointestinal and Abdominal Radiology
European Society of Gastrointestinal Endoscopy
European Society of Human Reproduction and Embryology
European Society of Intensive Care Medicine
European Society of Mastology
European Society of Neuroradiology
European Society of Paediatric Gastroenterology, Hepatology and Nutrition
European Society of Pediatric Otolaryngology—Head and Neck Surgery
European Society of Regional Anesthesia and Pain Therapy
European Society of Reproductive and Developmental Immunology
European Society of Residents in Urology
European Society of Sports Traumatology, Knee Surgery and Arthroscopy
European Society of Surgical Oncology
European Society of Thoracic Imaging
European Society of Urogenital Radiology
European Thyroid Association
European Union of General Practitioners
Extracorporeal Life Support Organization
FacioScapuloHumeral Muscular Dystrophy Society
Family Health International
Family Practice Association of Turkey
Federated Ambulatory Surgery Association
Federation of African Immunological Societies
Federation of European Cancer Societies
Federation of European Microbiological Societies
Federation of European Societies for Tropical Medicine and International Health
Fertility Society of Australia
Finnish Association of Physiotherapists
Finnish Cardiac Society
Finnish Diabetes Society
Finnish Medical Society Duodecim
Finnish Neuromuscular Disorders Association (Lihastautiliitto)
Finnish Neurosurgical Society
Finnish Society for Andrology
Finnish Society of Anaesthesiologists
Finnish Society of Community Physicians
Finnish Society of Periodontology

Florida Academy of Family Physicians
Florida Academy of Pain Medicine
Florida Allergy, Asthma and Immunology Society
Florida Association of Occupational and Environmental Medicine
Florida Association of Pediatric Cardiologists
Florida Association of Pediatric Critical Care Medicine
Florida Association of Pediatric Surgeons
Florida Dental Association
Florida Endocrine Society
Florida Gastroenterological Society
Florida Geriatrics Society
Florida Hospital Association
Florida Medical Association
Florida Neurosurgical Society
Florida Obstetric and Gynecologic Society
Florida Occupational Therapy Association
Florida Orthopaedic Society
Florida Pediatric Society
Florida Perfusion Society
Florida Physical Therapy Association
Florida Public Health Association
Florida Pulmonary Society
Florida Radiological Society
Florida Society for Adolescent Psychiatry
Florida Society for Histotechnology
Florida Society for Preventive Medicine
Florida Society for Respiratory Care
Florida Society of Anesthesiologists
Florida Society of Clinical Oncology
Florida Society of Colon and Rectal Surgeons
Florida Society of Dermatological Surgeons
Florida Society of Dermatology
Florida Society of Facial Plastic and Reconstructive Surgery
Florida Society of Internal Medicine
Florida Society of Neonatologists
Florida Society of Nephrology
Florida Society of Neurology
Florida Society of Ophthalmology
Florida Society of Otolaryngology
Florida Society of Pathologists
Florida Society of Pediatric Nephrologists
Florida Society of Physical Medicine and Rehabilitation

Florida Society of Plastic Surgeons
Florida Society of Psychiatry
Florida Society of Rheumatology
Florida Society of Thoracic and Cardiovascular Surgery
Florida Surgical Society
Florida Thoracic Society
Florida Urological Society
Florida Vascular Society
Flying Dentists Association
Flying Physicians Association
French Aviation and Medicine Society
French Federation of General Practitioners
French Society for Thoracic and Cardiovascular Surgery
French Society of Aesthetic Plastic Surgery
French Society of Neurosurgery
Gait and Clinical Movement Analysis Society
Genetics Society
Genetics Society of Japan
Genetics Society of Korea
Genetic Toxicology Association
Georgia Association of Emergency Medical Technicians
Georgia Association of Nurse Anesthetists
Georgia Dental Association
Georgia Medical Association
Georgia Orthopaedic Society
Georgia Pharmacy Association
Georgia Psychiatric Physicians Association
Georgia Public Health Association
Georgia Society for Respiratory Care
Georgia Thoracic Society
German Anatomical Society
German Dental Association
German Endocrine Society
German Epidemiological Society
German Medical Association
German Ophthalmological Society
German Sleep Society
German Society for Gynecological Endoscopy
German Society for Thoracic and Cardiovascular Surgery
German Society of Family Medicine
German Society of Neurosurgery
German Society of Orthodontists

German Society of Plastic Surgeons
German Society of Tropical Medicine and International Health
Greater Boston Physicians for Social Responsibility
Greek Association of General Practitioners
Greek-German Dental Association
Green Doctors—Ukranian Association of Doctors for the Environment
Guam Medical Society
Guild of Hospital Pharmacists
Haematology Society of Australia and New Zealand
Hans Popper Hepatopathology Society
Hawaii Academy of Family Physicians
Hawaii Dental Association
Hawaii Public Health Association
Healthcare Association of Hawaii
Healthcare Association of New York State
Heart Failure Society of America
Hellenic Aerospace Medical Society
Hellenic Cardiological Society
Hellenic Ophthalmological Society
Hellenic Radiological Society
Hellenic Society of Anaesthesiologists
Hellenic Society of Rheumatology
Hellenic Urological Association
Hemophilia Society
Hemophilia Society of Malaysia
Hip Society
Hispanic Dental Association
Holistic Dental Association
Hong Kong Academy of Medicine
Hong Kong Anti-Cancer Society
Hong Kong Association of Blood Transfusion and Haematology
Hong Kong Association of Dental Surgery Assistants
Hong Kong Association of Rehabilitation Medicine
Hong Kong Association of Sports Medicine and Sports Science
Hong Kong Cancer Chemotherapy Society
Hong Kong College of Anaesthesiologists
Hong Kong College of Cardiology
Hong Kong College of Emergency Medicine
Hong Kong College of Family Physicians
Hong Kong College of Obstetricians and Gynecologists
Hong Kong College of Paediatricians
Hong Kong College of Pathologists

Hong Kong College of Physicians
Hong Kong College of Psychiatrists
Hong Kong College of Radiologists
Hong Kong Dental Association
Hong Kong Geriatrics Society
Hong Kong Medical Association
Hong Kong Neurological Society
Hong Kong Neurosurgical Society
Hong Kong Nutrition Association
Hong Kong Occupational Safety and Health Association
Hong Kong Ophthalmological Society
Hong Kong Orthopaedic Association
Hong Kong Paediatric Haematology and Oncology Study Group
Hong Kong Paediatric Nephrology Society
Hong Kong Pediatric Society
Hong Kong Pharmacology Society
Hong Kong Physiotherapy Association
Hong Kong Prosthetic Dentistry Society
Hong Kong Society for Community Medicine
Hong Kong Society for Emergency Medicine and Surgery
Hong Kong Society for Immunology
Hong Kong Society for Infectious Diseases
Hong Kong Society of Critical Care Medicine
Hong Kong Society of Dermatology and Venereology
Hong Kong Society of Emergency Medicine and Surgery
Hong Kong Society of Gastroenterology
Hong Kong Society of Haematology
Hong Kong Society of Hospital Dentistry
Hong Kong Society of Minimal Access Surgery
Hong Kong Society of Nephrology
Hong Kong Society of Neurosciences
Hong Kong Society of Nuclear Medicine
Hong Kong Society of Palliative Medicine
Hong Kong Society of Periodontology
Hong Kong Society of Rheumatology
Hong Kong Society of Transplantation
Hong Kong Surgical Laser Association
Hong Kong Thoracic Society
Hong Kong Urological Association
Hospital Association of South Africa
Hospital Infection Society
Human Behavior and Evolution Society

Hungarian Medical Association
Hungarian Medical Association of America
Hungarian Neurosurgical Society
Hungarian Society for Angiology and Vascular Surgery
Hungarian Society for Immunology
Hungarian Society of Cardiology
Hydrocephalus Association
Hypertrophic Cardiomyopathy Association
Icelandic Heart Association
Icelandic Hemophilia Society
Idaho Academy of Family Physicians
Idaho Hospital Association
Idaho Medical Association
Idaho Primary Care Association
Idaho Society of Ophthalmology
Idaho State Dental Association
Illinois Academy of Family Physicians
Illinois College of Emergency Physicians
Illinois Dietetic Association
Illinois Public Health Association
Illinois Society for Respiratory Care
Illinois Society of Anesthesiologists
Illinois State Dental Society
Illinois State Perfusion Society
Immune Deficiency Foundation
Indian Academy of Cytologists
Indiana Dental Association
Indiana Dietetic Association
Indiana Occupational Therapy Association
Indiana Public Health Association
Indiana Society for Respiratory Care
Indiana State Medical Association
Indian Council of Medical Research
Indian Medical Association
Indian Pharmaceutical Congress Association
Indian Pharmacological Society
Indian Society of Critical Care Medicine
Indian Society of Extra-Corporeal Technology
Indonesian Society of Nephrology
Indonesian Society of Pediatricians
Infusion Nurses Society
Institute for Applied Behavioral Science

Institute for Applied Behavior Analysis
Institute for Preventive Sports Medicine
Institute of Food Technologists
Integrated Medicine Research Association
Intensive Care Society of Ireland
Interamerican College of Physicians and Surgeons
Inter-American Society of Hypertension
Internal Medicine Society of Australia and New Zealand
International Academy of Aviation and Space Medicine
International Academy of Classical Homeopathy
International Academy of Compounding Pharmacists
International Agency for Research on Cancer
International AIDS Society
International and American Associations of Clinical Nutritionists
International Arthroscopy Association
International Association for Cognitive Psychotherapy
International Association for Cross-Cultural Psychology
International Association for Disability and Oral Health
International Association for Orthodontics
International Association for the Study of Lung Cancer
International Association for the Study of Pain
International Association of Agricultural Medicine and Rural Health
International Association of Applied Psychology
International Association of Dento-Maxillo-Facial Radiology
International Association of Eating Disorder Professionals
International Association of EMTs and Paramedics
International Association of Endocrine Surgeons
International Association of Forensic Nurses
International Association of Group Psychotherapy
International Association of Military Flight Surgeon Pilots
International Association of Mind-Body Professionals
International Association of Physicians in Audiology
International Association of Sickle Cell Nurses and Physician Assistants
International Behavioral and Neural Genetics Society
International Behavioral Neuroscience Society
International Bone and Mineral Society
International Brain Research Organization
International Child Health Nursing Alliance
International Chiropractors Association
International Clinical Epidemiology Network
International College of Dentists
International College of Surgeons

International Congress of Oral Implantologists
International Council of Ophthalmology
International Council of Societies of Pathology
International Cystic Fibrosis Association
International Cytokine Society
International Epidemiological Association
International Federation for Cell Biology
International Federation of Gynecology and Obstetrics
International Federation of Pediatric and Adolescent Gynecology
International Flying Nurses Association
International Hospital Federation
International Lung Sounds Association
International Myeloma Foundation
International Neural Network Society
International Neuromodulation Society
International Neuropsychological Society
International Neurotoxicology Association
International Nursing Association for Clinical Simulation and Learning
International Pediatric Association
International Pediatric Endosurgery Group
International Pelvic Pain Society
International Perimetric Society
International Perinatal Doppler Society
International Proteolysis Society
International Psychoanalytic Association
International Psychogeriatric Association
International Psycho-Oncology Society
International Radiosurgery Support Association
International Rett Syndrome Association
International School Psychology Association
International Society for Adaptive Behavior
International Society for Antiviral Research
International Society for Applied Cardiovascular Biology
International Society for Autonomic Neuroscience
International Society for Behavioural Neuroscience
International Society for Clinical Biostatistics
International Society for Clinical Densitometry
International Society for Computer Aided Surgery
International Society for Cutaneous Lymphomas
International Society for Developmental and Comparative Immunology
International Society for Developmental Neuroscience
International Society for Developmental Psychobiology

International Society for Ecological Psychology
International Society for Environmental Epidemiology
International Society for Eye Research
International Society for Gynecological Endoscopy
International Society for Heart Research
International Society for Infectious Diseases
International Society for Interferon and Cytokine Research
International Society for Magnetic Resonance in Medicine
International Society for Minimally Invasive Cardiac Surgery
International Society for Neurochemistry
International Society for Neuropathology
International Society for Ocular Toxicology
International Society for Pediatric and Adolescent Diabetes
International Society for Peritoneal Dialysis
International Society for Plastination
International Society for Preventive Oncology
International Society for Prosthetics and Orthotics
International Society for Psychophysics
International Society for Quality in Health Care
International Society for Theoretical Psychology
International Society for the Study of Behavioral Development
International Society for the Study of Personal Relationships
International Society of Addiction Medicine
International Society of Andrology
International Society of Arthroscopy, Knee Surgery and Orthopaedic Sports Medicine
International Society of Biomechanics in Sports
International Society of Chemotherapy
International Society of Computerized Dentistry
International Society of Cyber Pathology
International Society of Developmental Biologists
International Society of Differentiation
International Society of Doctors for the Environment
International Society of Educators in Physiotherapy
International Society of Endocytobiology
International Society of Endovascular Specialists
International Society of Experimental Hematology
International Society of Exposure Analysis
International Society of Geographical and Epidemiological Ophthalmology
International Society of Gynecological Endocrinology
International Society of Gynecological Pathologists

International Society of Indoor Air Quality and Climate
International Society of Internal Medicine
International Society of Nephrology
International Society of Neuropathology
International Society of Political Psychology
International Society of Prenatal Diagnosis
International Society of Psychiatric Genetics
International Society of Psychoneuroendocrinology
International Society of Psychosomatic Obstetrics and Gynecology
International Society of Radiographers and Radiological Technologists
International Society of Radiology
International Society of Refractive Surgery
International Society of Surgery
International Society of Travel Medicine
International Society of Ultrasound in Obstetrics and Gynecology
International Society on Infant Studies
International Society on Thrombosis and Haemostasis
International Society on Toxinology
International Spinal Injection Society
International Transplant Coordinators Society
International Transplant Nurses Society
International Trauma Anesthesia and Critical Care Society
International Union of Biochemistry and Molecular Biology
International Union of Toxicology
Internet Dermatology Society
Internet Society of Orthopaedic Surgery and Trauma
Iowa Hospital Association
Iowa Medical Society
Iowa Physical Therapy Association
Iowa Public Health Association
Iowa Society of Periodontology
Irish Analytical Psychology Association
Irish Association of General Practitioners
Irish Cancer Society
Irish College of General Practitioners
Irish Diabetes Association
Irish Institute of Rural Health
Irish Kidney Association
Irish Medical Organization
Irish Nutrition and Dietetic Institute
Irish Society of Chartered Physiotherapists
Irish Society of Human Genetics

Irish Society of Obstetric Anesthesia
Irish Society of Occupational Medicine
Irish Society of Periodontology
Israel Aerospace Medicine Institute
Israel Association of Family Physicians
Israel Dental Association
Israel Dermatological Society
Israel Endocrine Society
Israel Gerontological Society
Israel Heart Society
Israeli Association for Emergency Medicine
Israel Immunological Society
Israeli Paramedics Association
Israeli Society for Allergy and Clinical Immunology
Israeli Society for Otolaryngology, Head and Neck Surgery
Israel Medical Association
Israel Orthopaedic Association
Israel Pediatric Endocrine Society
Israel Periodontal Society
Israel Society for Biological Psychiatry
Israel Society for Medical Mycology
Israel Society for Neurosciences
Israel Society for Occupational Therapy
Israel Society for Physiology and Pharmacology
Israel Society of Anaesthesiologists
Israel Society of Cardiothoracic Surgery
Israel Society of Hypertension
Israel Society of Oral Rehabilitation
Israel Society of Ultrasound in Obstetrics and Gynecology
Italian Academy of Family Physicians
Italian Academy of Rhinology
Italian Association of Hospital Cardiologists
Italian Society for Cardiac Surgery
Italian Society of Medical Andrology
Italian Society of Nephrology
Italian Society of Neurosurgery
Italian Society of Toxicology
Japan Academy of Neurosonology
Japan Association for International Health
Japan Association of Endocrine Surgeons
Japan Dental Association
Japan Dental Society of Oriental Medicine

Japan Endocrine Society
Japanese Academy of Family Medicine
Japanese Academy of Home Care Physicians
Japanese Academy of Occlusion and Health
Japanese Anatomical Association
Japanese Association for Molecular Target Therapy Cancer
Japanese Association for Surgery of Trauma
Japanese Association for Thoracic Surgery
Japanese Association of Cardiovascular Pharmacology
Japanese Association of Clinical Laboratory Physicians
Japanese Association of Endocrine Surgeons
Japanese Association of Rehabilitation Medicine
Japanese Association of School Health
Japanese Circulation Society
Japanese College of Cardiology
Japanese Coronary Association
Japanese Educational Clinical Cardiology Society
Japanese Gastric Cancer Association
Japanese Medical Society of Primary Care
Japanese Nursing Association
Japanese Ophthalmological Society
Japanese Orthodontic Society
Japanese Orthopaedic Association
Japanese Pharmacological Society
Japanese Physical Therapy Society
Japanese Psychiatric Nursing Association
Japanese Psychological Association
Japanese Society for Cardiovascular Surgery
Japanese Society for Dermatologic Surgery
Japanese Society for Immunology
Japanese Society for Intravascular Neurosurgery
Japanese Society for Jaw Deformities
Japanese Society for Minimally Invasive Orthopedic Surgery
Japanese Society for Oral and Maxillofacial Radiology
Japanese Society for Oral and Maxillofacial Surgery
Japanese Society for Pediatric Nephrology
Japanese Society for Pigment Cell Research
Japanese Society for Regenerative Medicine
Japanese Society for Therapeutic Radiology and Oncology
Japanese Society of Allergology
Japanese Society of Autogenic Therapy
Japanese Society of Cardiovascular Anesthesiologists

Japanese Society of Child Neurology
Japanese Society of Conservative Dentistry
Japanese Society of Gastroenterological Surgery
Japanese Society of Hematology
Japanese Society of Histocompatability and Immunogenetics
Japanese Society of Hypertension
Japanese Society of Intensive Care Medicine
Japanese Society of Internal Medicine
Japanese Society of Laboratory Medicine
Japanese Society of Magnetic Applications in Dentistry
Japanese Society of Medical Instrumentation
Japanese Society of Nephrology
Japanese Society of Neurology
Japanese Society of Neuropathology
Japanese Society of Nuclear Medicine
Japanese Society of Parasitology
Japanese Society of Pathology
Japanese Society of Pediatric Radiology
Japanese Society of Pediatric Surgeons
Japanese Society of Periodontology
Japanese Society of Radiological Technology
Japanese Society of Stomatognathic Function
Japanese Society of Tropical Medicine
Japanese Society of Ultrasonics in Medicine
Japan Medical Association
Japan Medical Society
Japan Neuroscience Society
Japan Pediatric Society
Japan Pharmaceutical Society
Japan Prosthodontic Society
Japan Radiological Society
Japan Society for Clinical Anesthesia
Japan Society for Lipid Nutrition
Japan Society for Magnetic Resonance in Medicine
Japan Society of Acupuncture and Moxibustion
Japan Society of Aerospace and Environmental Medicine
Japan Society of Anesthesiologists
Japan Society of Blood Transfusion
Japan Society of Chemotherapy
Japan Society of Clinical Oncology
Japan Society of Gene Therapy
Japan Society of Health Sciences

Japan Society of Hepatology
Japan Society of Obstetrics and Gynecology
Japan Society of Pain Clinicians
Japan Surgical Society
Kansas Academy of Family Physicians
Kansas Dental Association
Kansas Hospital Association
Kansas Medical Society
Kansas Physical Therapy Association
Kentucky Academy of Family Physicians
Kentucky Cardiopulmonary Rehabilitation Association
Kentucky Dental Association
Kentucky Medical Association
Kentucky Physical Therapy Association
Kentucky Psychiatric Association
Korean Association of Obstetricians and Gynecologists
Korean Dental Association
Korean Dermatological Association
Korean Diabetes Association
Korean Medical Association
Korean Ophthalmological Association
Korean Radiological Society
Korean Society for Cytopathology
Korean Society for Intravenous Anesthesia
Korean Society for Thoracic and Cardiovascular Surgery
Korean Society for Vascular Surgery
Korean Society of Anesthesiologists
Korean Society of Applied Pharmacology
Korean Society of Circulation
Korean Society of Clinical Pathologists
Korean Society of Infectious Diseases
Korean Society of Medical Genetics
Korean Society of Pharmacology
Latin American Thyroid Society
Lawson Wilkins Pediatric Endocrine Society
Lithuanian Heart Association
Louisiana Dental Association
Louisiana Hospital Association
Louisiana State Medical Society
Maine Academy of Family Physicians
Maine Association of Nurse Anesthetists
Maine Hospital Association

Maine Medical Association
Malaysian Dental Association
Malaysian Endocrine and Metabolic Society
Malaysian Endodontic Association
Malaysian Medical Association
Malaysian Urological Association
Malta Association of Physiotherapists
Malta College of Family Doctors
Manitoba College of Family Physicians
Manitoba Medical Association
Maryland Academy of Family Physicians
Maryland Dental Association
Maryland Dietetic Association
Maryland/District of Columbia Society for Respiratory Care
Maryland Hospital Association
Maryland Psychiatric Society
Maryland Public Health Association
Massachusetts College of Emergency Physicians
Massachusetts Dental Society
Massachusetts Hospital Association
Massachusetts Medical Society
Massachusetts Orthopaedic Association
Massachusetts Podiatric Medical Society
Massachusetts Public Health Association
Massachusetts Society for Respiratory Care
Massachusetts Society of Perfusion
Matrix Biology Society of Australia and New Zealand
Medical Association of South East Asian Nations
Medical Association of Thailand
Medical Group Management Association
Medical Oncology Group of Australia
Medical Research Council
Medical Review Officer Certification Council
Meningitis Foundation of America
Mexican Association of Plastic Surgery
Mexican College of Allergy, Asthma and Clinical Immunology
Mexican College of Pediatric Allergy, Asthma and Clinical Immunology
Mexican Society for Emergency Medicine
Mexican Society of Colon and Rectal Surgeons
Michigan Academy of Family Physicians
Michigan Association of Nurse Anesthetists
Michigan Association of Occupational Health Nurses

Michigan College of Emergency Physicians
Michigan Dental Association
Michigan Hospital Association
Michigan Podiatric Medical Society
Michigan Primary Care Association
Michigan Public Health Association
Michigan Society for Respiratory Care
Michigan State Medical Society
Microcirculatory Society
Mid America Orthopaedic Association
Mid Indiana Association of Occupational Health Nurses
Midwestern Vascular Surgical Society
Midwest Society for Pediatric Research
Midwest Teratology Association
Military Audiology Association
Military Dental Student Association
Minnesota Academy of Family Physicians
Minnesota Association of Cardiovascular and Pulmonary Rehabilitation
Minnesota Association of Periodontists
Minnesota Dental Association
Minnesota Hospital and Healthcare Partnership
Minnesota Psychiatric Society
Minnesota Public Health Association
Minnesota Society of Respiratory Care
Mississippi Hospital Association
Mississippi Public Health Association
Mississippi State Medical Association
Missouri Dental Association
Missouri Hospital Association
Missouri Medical Association
Missouri Society for Respiratory Care
Missouri State Orthopaedic Association
Montana Dental Association
Montana Medical Association
Montana Society for Respiratory Care
Montana Society of Anaesthesiologists
Movement Disorder Society
Muscular Dystrophy Italian Association
Nagoya Vascular Surgery Society
National Acupuncture Detoxification Association
National Adrenal Diseases Foundation
National Alaska Native American Indian Nurses Association

National Association for Biomedical Research
National Association for Chiropractic Medicine
National Association for Family Child Care
National Association for Healthcare Quality
National Association for Holistic Aromatherapy
National Association for Home Care
National Association for Public Health Statistics and Information Systems
National Association for the Advancement of Orthotics and Prosthetics
National Association for the Advancement of Psychoanalysis
National Association of Addiction Treatment Providers
National Association of Children's Hospitals and Related Institutions
National Association of Cognitive Behavioral Therapists
National Association of Dental Assistants
National Association of Dental Laboratories
National Association of Health Data Organizations
National Association of Hispanic Nurses
National Association of Hospital Hospitality Houses
National Association of Physicians for the Environment
National Association of Psychiatric Health Systems
National Association of Rehabilitation Providers and Agencies
National Association of State Alcohol and Drug Abuse Directors
National Association of Theatre Nurses
National Black Nurses Association
National Board for Certification in Occupational Therapy
National Board of Chiropractic Examiners
National Board of Forensic Chiropractors
National Brain Tumor Radiosurgery Association
National Childhood Cancer Foundation
National College of Naturopathic Medicine
National Dysautonomia Research Foundation
National Emergency Medical Association
National EMS Pilots Association
National Enuresis Society
National Family Caregivers Association
National Federation of Licensed Practical Nurses
National Flight Paramedics Association
National Foundation of Ectodermal Dysplasia
National Hemophilia Foundation
National Keratoconus Foundation
National Med-Peds Residents' Association
National Neurofibromatosis Foundation
National Neurotrauma Society

National Perinatal Association
National Psoriasis Foundation
National Rehabilitation Association
National Rosacea Society
National Spasmodic Torticollis Association
National Spinal Cord Injury Association
National Stroke Association
National Tuberous Sclerosis Association
National Tumor Registrars Association
National Vulvodynia Association
Navy Anesthesia Society
Nebraska Academy of Family Physicians
Nebraska Hospital Association
Nebraska Physical Therapy Association
Nebraska Public Health Association
Nebraska Society for Respiratory Care
Neonatal and Paediatric Pharmacists Group
Nephrogenic Diabetes Insipidus Foundation
Netherlands Aeromedical Institute
Netherlands Association for Cardio-Thoracic Surgery
Netherlands Epidemiological Society
Netherlands Hemophilia Society
Netherlands Patient Organization for Primary Immunodeficiencies
Netherlands Society for Parasitology
Netherlands Society of Neurosurgeons
Netherlands Society of Plastic Surgery
Netherlands Society of Tropical Medicine
Neuropathy Association
Nevada Academy of Family Physicians
Nevada Dental Association
Nevada Physical Therapy Association
New England Society for Vascular Surgery
New England Society of Anesthesiologists
New England Society of Plastic and Reconstructive Surgery
New Hampshire Medical Society
New Jersey Academy of Family Physicians
New Jersey Academy of Otolaryngology
New Jersey Association of Nurse Anesthetists
New Jersey Dental Association
New Jersey Hospital Association
New Jersey Medical Society
New Jersey Psychiatric Association

New Jersey Public Health Association
New Jersey Speech-Language and Hearing Association
New Jersey State Perfusion Society
New Mexico Academy of Family Physicians
New Mexico Allergy Society
New Mexico Hospitals and Health Systems Association
New Mexico Medical Society
New Mexico Public Health Association
New Mexico Society for Respiratory Care
New York Academy of Family Physicians
New York Physical Therapy Association
New York State Dental Association
New York State Occupational Therapy Association
New York State Ophthalmological Society
New York State Psychiatric Association
New York State Radiological Society
New York State Society for Respiratory Care
New York State Society of Anesthesiology
New York State Society of Orthopaedic Surgeons
New Zealand Dental Association
New Zealand Medical Association
New Zealand Microbiological Society
New Zealand Psychological Society
New Zealand Society of Otolaryngology Head and Neck Surgery
New Zealand Society of Podiatrists
New Zealand Society of Vascular Surgery
Nordic Association for Andrology
Nordic Orthopedic Federation
North American Nursing Diagnosis Association
North American Society for Cardiac Imaging
North American Society for Pediatric and Adolescent Gynecology
North American Society for Pediatric Exercise Medicine
North American Society for Pediatric Gastroenterology, Hepatology and Nutrition
North American Society of Homeopaths
North Carolina Academy of Family Physicians
North Carolina Anesthesia Practice Management Association
North Carolina Association of Nurse Anesthetists
North Carolina Association of Occupational Health Nurses
North Carolina Dental Society
North Carolina Medical Society
North Carolina Physical Therapy Association

North Carolina Society for Respiratory Care
North Carolina Society of Anesthesiologists
North Dakota Association of Nurse Anesthetists
North Dakota Healthcare Association
North Dakota Public Health Association
Northern Ireland Society for Computing in Anesthesia
Northern Ireland Society of Anaesthesiologists
Northern Virginia Association of Occupational Health Nurses
Northwest Academy of Otolaryngology
Northwest Association of Cardiovascular and Pulmonary Rehabilitation
Northwest Association of Occupational and Environmental Medicine
Northwest Territories Medical Association
Norwegian Anaesthesiological Society
Norwegian Council on Cardiovascular Diseases
Norwegian Hemophilia Society
Norwegian Medical Association
Nova Scotia Medical Society
Nutrition Society
Obesity Surgery Society of Australia and New Zealand
Obstetric Anaesthetists Association
Obstetric and Gynecological Society of Singapore
Occupational and Environmental Medical Association of Canada
Occupational Injury Prevention and Rehabilitation Society
Ohio Academy of General Dentistry
Ohio Dental Association
Ohio Dietetic Association
Ohio Occupational Therapy Association
Ohio Pharmacists Association
Ohio Physical Therapy Association
Ohio Podiatric Medical Association
Ohio Psychiatric Association
Ohio Public Health Association
Ohio Society for Respiratory Care
Ohio State Medical Association
Ohio State Radiological Society
Oklahoma Dental Association
Oklahoma Hospital Association
Oklahoma Podiatric Medical Association
Oklahoma Psychiatric Physicians Association
Oklahoma Society of Certified Perfusionists
Oklahoma State Medical Association
Oncology Nursing Society

Ontario Academy of General Dentistry
Ontario Association of Orthodontists
Ontario Dental Association
Ontario Pediatric Association
Ontario Physical Therapy Association
Ontario Podiatric Medical Association
Ophthalmic Anesthesia Society
Oregon Association of Nurse Anesthetists
Oregon Dental Association
Oregon Diabetes Educators
Oregon Medical Association
Oregon Primary Care Association
Oregon Public Health Association
Oregon Radiological Society
Oregon Society for Respiratory Care
Oregon Society of Health System Pharmacists
Organization for Safety and Asepsis Procedures
Orthopaedic Research and Education Foundation
Orthopaedic Research Society
Orthopaedic Trauma Society
Osteoarthritis Research Society
Otolaryngological Society of Japan
Otorhinolaryngological Research Society
Pacific Coast Society of Orthodontists
Pacific Society for Reproductive Health
Pakistan Society for the Study of Pain
Pakistan Society of Gastroenterology
Pan American Aerobiology Association
Pan American Association for Biochemistry and Molecular Biology
Pan American Association of Anatomists
Pan American Association of Ophthalmology
Pan American Health Association
Pan American Society for Clinical Virology
Pathological Society of Great Britain and Ireland
Pediatric/Adolescent Gastroesophageal Reflux Association
Pediatric Association of Bosnia/Herzegovina
Pediatric Endocrinology Nursing Society
Pediatric Infectious Disease Society
Pediatric Orthopaedic Society of North America
Pennsylvania Academy of General Dentistry
Pennsylvania Dental Association
Pennsylvania Medical Society

Pennsylvania Orthopaedic Society
Pennsylvania Perfusion Society
Pennsylvania Public Health Association
Peripheral Vascular Surgery Society
Peruvian American Medical Society
Pharmaceutical Society of Hong Kong
Pharmacy Guild of Australia
Philippine Academy of General Dentistry
Philippine Academy of Ophthalmology
Philippine Association of Thoracic and Cardiovascular Surgeons
Philippine Cancer Society
Philippine College of Physicians
Philippine College of Surgeons
Philippine Dermatological Association
Philippine Heart Association
Philippine Medical Association
Philippine Neurological Association
Philippine Orthopedic Association
Philippine Pediatric Society
Philippine Psychiatric Association
Philippine Society of Anaesthesiologists
Philippine Society of Climacteric Medicine
Philippine Society of Gastroenterology
Philippine Society of General Surgeons
Philippine Society of Oncologists
Philippine Society of Pediatric Surgeons
Philippine Urological Association
Physicians for Social Responsibility
Physiological Society
Polish Society of Anaesthesiologists
Portuguese Association of General Practitioners
Primary Immunodeficiency Association
Professional Association of Belgian Cardiologists
Public Health Association of Nebraska
Puerto Rico Association of Pediatric Surgeons
Quebec Urological Association
Renal Association
Rhode Island Dental Association
Rhode Island Medical Society
Rocky Mountain Cardiopulmonary Rehabilitation Association
Romanian Society of Neurosurgery
Royal Australasian College of Dental Surgeons

Royal Australasian College of Medical Administrators
Royal Australian and New Zealand College of Obstetricians and Gynecologists
Royal College of Anaesthetists
Royal College of Anesthesiologists of Thailand
Royal College of Dentists of Canada
Royal College of Ophthalmologists
Royal College of Pathologists
Royal College of Pediatrics and Child Health
Royal College of Physicians and Surgeons of Glasgow
Royal College of Physicians of Edinburgh
Royal College of Radiologists
Royal College of Surgeons in Ireland
Royal College of Surgeons of Edinburgh
Royal College of Surgeons of England
Royal Microscopic Society
Royal New Zealand College of General Practitioners
Royal Pharmaceutical Society of Great Britain
Royal Society for the Promotion of Health
Royal Society of Medicine
Royal Society of Tropical Medicine and Hygiene
Rural Doctors Association of Australia
Russian Public Health Association
Russian Scientific Society of Cardiology
Russian Society of Immunology
Saskatchewan Medical Association
Scleroderma Federation
Scleroderma Foundation
Scoliosis Association
Scottish Committee for Orthopaedics and Trauma
Scottish Intensive Care Society
Scottish Microbiology Society
Singapore Cancer Society
Singapore Dental Association
Singapore Medical Association
Sjogren's Syndrome Foundation
Slovak Society of Anesthesia and Intensive Care
Slovenian Society of Cardiology
Society for Ambulatory Anesthesia
Society for Anaerobic Microbiology
Society for Applied Microbiology
Society for a Science of Clinical Psychology

Society for Behavioral Neuroendocrinology
Society for Biomaterials
Society for Cardiac Angiography and Interventions
Society for Cardiological Science and Technology
Society for Cardiovascular and Interventional Radiology
Society for Cardiovascular Magnetic Resonance
Society for Cardiovascular Pathology
Society for Clinical Trials
Society for Computer Applications in Radiology
Society for Computing and Technology in Anesthesia
Society for Consumer Psychology
Society for Developmental and Behavioral Pediatrics
Society for Endocrinology
Society for Epidemiological Research
Society for Experimental Biology
Society for Fetal Urology
Society for Health Services Research in Radiology
Society for Heart Valve Disease
Society for Hematopathology
Society for Industrial Microbiology
Society for Intravenous Anesthesia
Society for Investigative Dermatology
Society for Light Treatment and Biological Rhythms
Society for Mathematical Psychology
Society for Mucosal Immunology
Society for Neuroscience
Society for Neurosurgical Anesthesia and Critical Care
Society for Obstetric Anesthesia and Perinatology
Society for Occupational and Environmental Health
Society for Office Based Anesthesia
Society for Pediatric and Perinatal Epidemiologic Research
Society for Pediatric Anesthesia
Society for Pediatric Dermatology
Society for Pediatric Pathology
Society for Pediatric Radiology
Society for Pediatric Urology
Society for Personality and Social Psychology
Society for Police and Criminal Psychology
Society for Prevention Research
Society for Progressive Supranuclear Palsy
Society for Psychophysiological Research
Society for Psychotherapy Research

Society for Research in Adult Development
Society for Research in Child Development
Society for Sex Therapy Research
Society for Social Medicine
Society for Surgery of the Alimentary Tract
Society for Teachers of Family Medicine
Society for Technology in Anesthesia
Society for the Exploration of Psychotherapy Integration
Society for the Study of Addiction
Society for the Study of Ingestive Behavior
Society for Ultrastructure Pathology
Society of Anaesthetists of Hong Kong
Society of Behavioral Medicine
Society of Biological Psychiatry
Society of Breast Imaging
Society of British Neurological Surgeons
Society of Cardiothoracic Surgeons of Great Britain and Ireland
Society of Cardiovascular Anesthesiologists
Society of Clinical Psychiatrists UK
Society of Computed Body Tomography and Magnetic Resonance
Society of Forensic Toxicology
Society of Gastrointestinal Radiologists
Society of General Physiologists
Society of Industrial and Organizational Psychology
Society of Laparendoscopic Surgeons
Society of Military Orthopaedic Surgeons
Society of Nuclear Medicine
Society of Occupational Medicine
Society of Otolaryngology and Head-Neck Nurses
Society of Perfusionists of Great Britain and Ireland
Society of Radiologists in Ultrasound
Society of Rural Physicians of Canada
Society of Skeletal Radiology
Society of Surgical Oncology
Society of Thoracic Radiology
Society of Toxicologic Pathology
Society of Toxicology Canada
Society of Trauma Nurses
Society of Urologic Nurses and Associates
Society of Uroradiology
Society of U.S. Air Force Flight Surgeons
Society of U.S. Army Flight Surgeons

Society of U.S. Naval Flight Surgeons
Society of Vascular Technology
South African Critical Care Society
South African Dental Association
South African Medical Association
South African Orthopaedic Association
South African Pulmonology Society
South African Society of Anaesthesiologists
South Carolina Dental Association
South Carolina Hospital Association
South Carolina Medical Association
South Dakota State Medical Association
Southern Academy of Periodontology
Southern Association for Primary Care
Southern California Public Health Association
Southern Medical Association
Southern Orthopaedic Association
Southern Society for Pediatric Research
Southern Thoracic Surgical Association
Spanish Society of Anatomy
Spanish Society of Neurosurgery
Spondylitis Association of America
Sudden Infant Death Syndrome Alliance
Surgical Infection Society
Swedish Association of Cardiothoracic Surgery
Swedish Dental Association
Swedish Medical Association
Swedish Orthopaedic Association
Swedish Society for Vascular Surgery
Swedish Society of Cardiology
Swedish Society of Gastroenterology
Swiss Anesthesia Society
Swiss Medical Association
Swiss Society for Anatomy, Histology and Embryology
Swiss Society for Vascular Surgery
Swiss Society of Cardiology
Swiss Society of Pharmacology and Toxicology
Tennessee Dental Association
Tennessee Medical Association
Tennessee Perfusion Association
Tennessee Primary Care Association
Tennessee Public Health Association

Texas Academy of Family Physicians
Texas Dental Association
Texas Dietetic Association
Texas Health Care Association
Texas Hospital Association
Texas Medical Association
Texas Orthopaedic Association
Texas Osteopathic Medical Association
Texas Pain Society
Texas Physical Therapy Association
Texas Psychological Association
Texas Public Health Association
Texas Radiological Society
Texas Society of Anesthesiologists
Texas Society of Pathologists
Thailand Dental Association
Thailand Dermatological Association
Thailand Medical Association
Thailand Neurosurgical Association
Thailand Occupational Medicine Association
Thailand Orthodontic Society
Thailand Trauma Association
Thailand Urological Association
Thoracic Surgery Directors Association
Thoracic Surgery Residents Association
Thyroid Federation International
Thyroid Foundation of America
Transplantation Society
Trauma Association of Canada
Trigeminal Neuralgia Association
Turkish Pharmacological Society
Turkish Radiological Society
Turkish Society of Anaesthesiologists
Turkish Society of Clinical Neurophysiology, EEG-EMG
Turkish Society of Toxicology
Turner's Syndrome Society
United Kingdom Genetical Society
United Mitochondrial Disease Foundation
United States and Canadian Academy of Pathology
Urological Society of Australasia
Urological Society of India
U.S. Army Aviation Medicine Association

Utah Medical Association
Utah Pharmaceutical Association
Utah Podiatric Medical Association
Utah Public Health Association
Utah Radiological Society
Vascular Society of India
Vermont Academy of Family Physicians
Vermont Association of Hospitals and Health Systems
Vermont State Dental Society
Vietnam General Association of Medicine and Pharmacy
Virginia Academy of Family Physicians
Virginia Association of Cardiovascular and Pulmonary Rehabilitation
Virginia Dental Association
Virginia Infectious Disease Society
Virginia Medical Society
Virginia Orthopaedic Society
Virginia Perfusion Society
Virginia Pharmacists Association
Virginia Podiatric Medical Association
Virginia Primary Care Association
Virginia State Association of Occupational Health Nurses
Visiting Nurses Association of America
Washington Academy of Family Physicians
Washington State Chiropractic Association
Washington State Dental Association
Washington State Hospital Association
Washington State Radiological Society
Western Orthopedic Association
Western Pacific Association of Critical Care Medicine
Western Psychological Association
Western Society for Pediatric Research
West Virginia Public Health Association
West Virginia State Medical Association
Wilderness Medical Society
Wilson's Disease Association
Wisconsin Academy of Family Physicians
Wisconsin Health and Hospital Association
Wisconsin Perfusion Society
Wisconsin Primary Health Care Association
Wisconsin Society for Cardiovascular and Pulmonary Rehabilitation
World Association of Family Doctors
World Council of Optometry

World Federation of Orthodontists
World Heart Federation
World Hypertension League
Wyoming Medical Society
Yukon Medical Association

Appendix B

Bibliography of Position Document Literature

American Academy of Allergy (1981). American Academy of Allergy: Position statements: Controversial techniques. *J. Allergy Clin. Immunol.* 67(5): 333-338.

American Association of Dental Schools (1980). Proceedings of the 57th annual session: Appendix A—Policy statements and position papers. *J. Dent. Educ.* 44(7): 413-426.

American Association of Occupational Health Nurses (AAOHN) (1986). AAOHN position statements. *AAOHN J.* 34(4): 178-184.

American Health Information Management Association (1993). American Health Information Management Association: Position statement. Issue: Position statements. *J. AHIMA* 64(11): 105.

American Nephrology Nurses Association (ANNA) (1995). ANNA position statements. *ANNA J.* 22(3): 269-274.

American Nephrology Nurses Association (ANNA) (1996). ANNA position statements. *ANNA J.* 23(2): 163-170.

American Nephrology Nurses Association (ANNA) (1997). ANNA position statements. *ANNA J.* 24(2): 180-188.

American Nephrology Nurses Association (ANNA) (1998). ANNA position statements. *ANNA J.* 25(2): 179-181.

American Nurses Association (1988). Ethics and nursing: Position statements and guidelines. *ANA Publ.* G-175: 1-16.

American Nurses Association (1992). Compendium of position statements on the nurse's role in end-of-life decisions: American Nurses Association Center for Ethics and Human Rights task force on the nurse's role in end-of-life decisions. *ANA Publ.* 9: 1-13.

American Public Health Association (2001). Policy statements adopted by the governing council of the American Public Health Association, November 15, 2000. *Am. J. Public Health* 91(3): 476-521.

American Public Health Association (1998). Policy statements adopted by the governing council of the American Public Health Association, November 18, 1998. *Am. J. Public Health* 89(3): 428-450.

American Speech-Language-Hearing Association (ASHA) (1991). Draft position statements and guidelines: Balance system assessment. *ASHA* 33(5): 58-59.

American Speech-Language-Hearing Association (ASHA) (1996). Reference list: Position statement, guidelines, and other relevant papers. *ASHA* Suppl. 38(2 Suppl. 16): 64-66.

American Speech-Language-Hearing Association (ASHA) (1999). Reference list: Position statements, guidelines, and other relevant papers. *ASHA* Suppl. 41(2 Suppl. 19): 47-49.

Association of Perioperative Registered Nurses (AORN) (2002). AORN position statements and resolution adopted. *Plast. Surg. Nurs.* 22(4): 181-184.

Barr, P., Pinch, W.J., and Boardman, K. (1993). Focus on ethics: ANA issues position statements. *Nebr. Nurse* 26(1): 21-22.

Bloom, S.P. (1983). Policy and procedure statements that communicate. *Pers. J.* 62(9): 711-718.

Clifford, T.L. (2003). An introduction to ASPAN's 2003 position statements. *J. Perianesth. Nurs.* 18(5): 298-300.

Compendium of position statements, guidelines and consensus statements on allergic and immunological diseases (2001). *Ann. Allergy Asthma Immunol.* 87(2 Suppl. 2): 1-31.

Council on Dental Research (1975). Position statements from the Council on Dental Research. *J. Am. Dent. Assoc.* 91(6): 1253-1254.

Curtiss, C.P. (2004). Consensus statements, positions, standards, and guidelines for pain and care at the end of life. *Semin. Oncol. Nurs.* 20(2): 121-139.

Emergency Nurses Association (1988). Emergency Nurses Association position statements. *J. Emerg. Nurs.* 14(4): 29A-32A.

Fain, J.A. (2003). Position statements, technical reviews, and white papers: Understanding the differences. *Diabetes Educ.* 29(6): 880-881.

Fain, J.A. (2003). Understanding the meaning of position statements. *Diabetes Educ.* 28(5): 650.

Gear, A.J. and Edlich, R.F. (1996). Mission statements: Guidelines for principles medical leadership. *Acad. Emerg. Med.* 3(8): 801-803.

Gilbert, T.T. and Taylor, J.S. (1999). How to evaluate and implement clinical policies. *Fam. Pract. Manag.* 6(3): 28-33.

Glover, P. (2000). Midwifery policies, position statements, and standards: How do we know that we meet them? *Aust. Coll. Midwives* 13(1): 3-4.

Gorenberg, B.D., Alderman, M.C., and Cruise, M.J. (1991). Social policy statements: Guidelines for decision making. *Int. Nurs. Rev.* 38(1): 11-13.

Gunn, J. (2004). The Royal College of Psychiatrists and the death penalty. *J. Am. Acad. Psychiatry Law* 32(2): 188-191.

Haas, L.B. (1990). The role and importance of position statements. *Diabetes Educ.* 16(3): 172.

Haylock, P.J. (2004). Position statements: Advocacy or futility? *Semin. Oncol. Nurs.* 20(2): 71-73.

Jefferson, R. (2001). Critical thinking: Position statements: Professional tool to support today's nurses. *Dynamics* 12(1): 4-5.

Jekel, J.F. (1991). Health departments in the US 1920-1988: Statements of mission with special reference to the role of C.-E.A. Winslow. *Yale J. Biol. Med.* 64(5): 467-479.

Katz, D.L. and Lane, D.S. (2002). Guidance at the many edges of evidence: Position statements of the American College of Preventive Medicine. *Am. J. Prev. Med.* 23(4): 312-313.

Katz, P.R. and Ouslander, J.G. (1996). Clinical practice guidelines and position statements: The American Geriatrics Society approach. *J. Am. Geriatr. Soc.* 44(9): 1123-1124.

Leib, E.S., Lenchik, L., Bilezikian, J.P., Maricic, M.J., and Watts, N.B. (2002). Position statements of the International Society for Clinical Densitometry: Methodology. *J. Clin. Densitom.* 5 Suppl: S5-S10.

Leigh, J. (1987). The CLD position statements: Development and purpose. *J. Learn Disabil.* 20(6): 347-350.

Loescher, L. (2004). Nursing roles in cancer prevention position statements. *Semin. Oncol. Nurs.* 20(2): 111-120.

Lohr, K.N., Eleazer, K., and Mauskopf, J. (1998). Health policy issues and applications for evidence-based medicine and clinical practice guidelines. *Health Policy* 46(1). 1-19.

National Association of Neonatal Nurses (NANN) (1995). NANN board of directors approves position statements. *Neonatal Netw.* 14(5): 52-55.

National Association of Pediatric Nurse Practitioners (NAPNAP) (1992). NAPNAP position statements. *J. Pediatr. Health Care* 6(4): 226.

National League for Nursing (NLN) (1982). NLN position statements. *NLN Publ.* 41(189): 1-33.

National Mental Health Association (NMHA) (1970). NMHA position statements on family life and sex education and marriage counselors. *Ment. Hyg.* 54(4): 591-592.

Policy statements (1999). *Ann. Emerg. Med.* 34(4): 576-578.

Polosa, R., Cacciola, R.R., Avanzi, G.C., and DiMaria, G.U. (2002). Making, disseminating and using clinical guidelines. *Monaldi Arch. Chest Dis.* 57(1): 44-47.

President's message: Stepping out: Issuing position statements to inform health policy (2000). *Nurs. Outlook* 48(1): 40-41.

Quill, T.E. and Cassel, C.K. (2003). Professional organizations position statements on physician assisted suicide: A case studied for neutrality. *Ann. Intern. Med.* 138(3): 208-211.

Renvoize, E.B., Hampshaw, S.M., Pinder, J.M., and Ayres, P. (1997). What are hospitals doing about clinical guidelines? *Qual. Health Care* 6(4): 187-191.

Service, F.J., Rizza, R.A., and Zimmerman, B.R. (1987). Comment on position statements. *Diabetes Care* 10(3): 374-375.

Society for Vascular Nursing (1994). SVN issues position statements. *J. Vasc. Nurs.* 12(1): 27-28.

Squires, B.P. (1991). Statements from professional associations, specialty groups and consensus conferences: What editors expect. *CMAJ* 145(4): 297-298.

Strayer, A.H. (1996). Society of Infectious Diseases pharmacist position papers. *Pharm. Pract. Manag. Q.* 16(2): 62-65.

Transcultural Nursing Society (1998). Policy statements to guide transcultural nursing standards and practices. *J. Transcult. Nurs.* 9(2): 75-77.

Wienke, K. (1991). Specialty nurses organizations develop position statements. *Orthop. Nurs.* 10(6): 6-7.

Woolf, S.H., Patrick, K., and Scutchfield, F.D. (1996). Taking a seat at the table: The new practice policy statements of the American College of Preventive Medicine. *Am. J. Prev. Med.* 12(5): 338-339.

World Medical Association (1996). World Medical Association adopts statements, etc. on miscellaneous matters. *Int. Dig. Health Legis.* 47(1): 100-107.

World Medical Association (1997). World Medical Association adopts statements, etc. on miscellaneous matters. *Int. Dig. Health Legis.* 48(1): 92-97.

References

Ambulatory Pediatric Association (2001). *Policy on policies: Guidelines for policy statement development.* McLean, VA: Author.

British Toxicology Society (n.d.). *The production of position statements and position papers.* Macclesfield, UK: Author.

Campbell, A. and Huxtable, R. (2003). The position statement and its commentators: Consensus, compromise or confusion? *Palliative Medicine* 17: 180-183.

Clangy, M.J. (2001). Position statements. *Emergency Medicine Journal* 18(5): 329.

International Nurses Society on Addictions (1999). Guidelines for position papers. Obtained online at <http://www.intnsa.org>.

International Pharmaceutical Federation (2001). Definitions of the different types of FIP documents. Obtained online at <http://www.fip.org>.

Leib, E.S., Lenchik, L., Bilezikian, J.P., Maricic, M.J., and Watts, N.B. (2002). Position statements of the International Society for Clinical Densitometry: Methodology. *Journal of Clinical Densitometry* 5(Suppl. 3): 5-10.

Leigh, J. (1987). The CLD position statements: Development and purpose. *Journal of Learning Disabilities* 20(6): 347-348.

National Association of County and City Health Officials (1998). NACCHO policy development process. Obtained online at <http://www.naccho.org>.

National Guideline Clearinghouse (1999). Inclusion critiera: Definition of clinical practice guideline. Obtained online at <http://www.guideline.gov>.

Pennsylvania Medical Society (2000). Memo on resolutions. Obtained online at <http://www.amwa-doc.org>.

Society for Neuroscience (1999). Guidelines: Responsible conduct regarding scientific communication. Obtained online at <http://www.sfn.org>.

Society for Public Health Education (1982). SOPHE resolutions policy and procedures. Obtained online at <http://www.sophe.org>.

Strayer, A.H. (1996). Society of Infectious Diseases Pharmacists (SIDP) position papers. *Pharmacy Practice Management Quarterly* 16(2): 62-65.

Index

Haworth Medical Information Sources
Sandra Wood, MLS, MBA
Senior Editor

BIOMEDICAL ORGANIZATIONS: A WORLDWIDE GUIDE TO POSITION DOCUMENTS by Dale A. Stirling. (2006).

MEDICAL LIBRARY DOWNSIZING: ADMINISTRATIVE, PROFESSIONAL, AND PERSONAL STRATEGIES FOR COPING WITH CHANGE by Michael J. Schott. (2005). "Michael Schott is fresh, funny, and fearless in this take-no-prisoners guide to dealing with corporate takeovers, mergers, and downsizing that threaten and challenge the survival of hospital libraries." *Elizabeth Connor, MLS, AHIP, Assistant Professor of Library Science, The Citadel, Charleston, South Carolina*

THE HERBAL INTERNET COMPANION: HERBS AND HERBAL MEDICINE ONLINE by David J. Owen. (2002). "Finally, someone has written a concise, referenced, unbiased, and thorough guide to navigating the Internet for information on herbs. This book is knowledgeable and factual, avoiding hyperbole, and plunging straight for the truth. . . . I consider this book an absolute must for anyone, professional or lay, seeking meaningful sources of herbal information on the Internet." *Paul L. Schiff Jr., PhD, Professor of Pharmaceutical Sciences, University of Pittsburgh*

HEALTH CARE RESOURCES ON THE INTERNET: A GUIDE FOR LIBRARIANS AND HEALTH CARE CONSUMERS edited by M. Sandra Wood. (2000). "A practical guide and an essential research tool to the Internet's vast and varied resources for health care has arrived—and its voice is professional and accessible . . . This comprehensive work is an important reference tool that is readable and enjoyable." *Elizabeth (Betty) R. Warner, MSLS, AHIP, Coordinator of Information Literacy Programs, Academic Information Services and Research, Thomas Jefferson University, Philadelphia, Pennsylvania*

EATING POSITIVE: A NUTRITION GUIDE AND RECIPE BOOK FOR PEOPLE WITH HIV/AIDS by Jeffrey T. Huber and Kris Riddlesperger. (1998). "Four stars! . . . A much-needed book that could have a positive impact on the quality of life for persons with HIV/AIDS. . . . Many of the recipes are old favorites that have been enhanced for the person with HIV. . . . All people with nutritional problems may also find this book helpful. It is not reserved solely for the person with HIV/AIDS." *Doody Publishing, Inc.*

HIV/AIDS AND HIV/AIDS-RELATED TERMINOLOGY: A MEANS OF ORGANIZING THE BODY OF KNOWLEDGE by Jeffrey T. Huber and Mary L. Gillaspy. (1996). "Provides the needed standardized terminology to describe large HIV/AIDS collections. . . . A welcome book for any cataloger, indexer, or archivist who is faced with organizing a mass of information that is growing very rapidly. . . . highly recommended for all librarians with extensive collections." *Booklist: Reference Books Bulletin*

HIV/AIDS COMMUNITY INFORMATION SERVICES: EXPERIENCES IN SERVING BOTH AT-RISK AND HIV-INFECTED POPULATIONS by Jeffrey T. Huber. (1996). "Provides a well-organized introduction to HIV/AIDS information services that will be useful to those affected by HIV disease, health care practitioners, librarians, and other information professionals. Appropriate for all libraries and an excellent reference resource." *CHOICE*

USER EDUCATION IN HEALTH SCIENCES LIBRARIES: A READER edited by M. Sandra Wood. (1995). "A welcome addition to any health sciences library collection. A valuable tool for both academic and hospital librarians, as well as library school students interested in bibliographic instruction." *National Network*

CD-ROM IMPLEMENTATION AND NETWORKING IN HEALTH SCIENCES LIBRARIES edited by M. Sandra Wood. (1993). "Neatly compacts information about the history, selection, and management of CD-ROM technology in libraries. . . . Librarians at all levels of CD-ROM implementation can benefit from the solutions and ideas presented." *Bulletin of the Medical Library Association*

HOW TO FIND INFORMATION ABOUT AIDS, SECOND EDITION edited by Jeffrey T. Huber. (1992). "Since organizations and sources in this field are constantly changing, this updated edition is welcome. . . . A valuable resource for health or medical and public library collections." *Booklist: Reference Books Bulletin*

Printed in the United States
by Baker & Taylor Publisher Services